WORKBOOK
to Accompany

ENDING
SPOUSE / PARTNER ABUSE

Robert Geffner, PhD, ABPN, is the Founder and President of the Family Violence and Sexual Assault Institute now located in Fort Worth, TX, and San Diego, CA, he is a Licensed Psychologist and a Licensed Marriage, Family & Child Counselor who was the clinical director of a large private-practice mental health clinic in Texas for 15 years, and is a former Professor of Psychology at the University of Texas at Tyler. Dr. Geffner is currently a Clinical Research Professor of Psychology at the California School of Professional Psychology in San Diego. He is also the editor of the *Journal of Child Sexual Abuse, Aggression, Maltreatment & Trauma,* and the *Family Violence & Sexual Assault Bulletin,* and co-editor of the *Journal of Emotional Abuse,* all internationally disseminated. He has a doctorate in psychology and postdoctorate training in clinical psychology, neuropsychology, child psychology, family violence, child maltreatment, forensic psychology, and diagnostic assessment. He has a Diplomate in Clinical Neuropsychology from the American Board of Professional Neuropsychology. He has served as an adjunct faculty member for the National Judicial College since 1990. His publications include treatment manuals and books concerning family violence, and numerous book chapters and journal articles concerning spouse/partner abuse, child abuse, child psychology, forensic issues, neuropsychology and psychological assessment. He has served as a consultant and grant reviewer for the National Center for Child Abuse and Neglect, the Department of Health and Human Services, the National Institutes of Mental Health, and other national and state agencies, and has served on various national and state committees dealing with various aspects of family psychology, family violence, and child abuse. He was a founding member and former President of the Board of the East Texas Crisis Center and Shelter for Battered Women and their Children in Tyler, TX. He has been involved in teaching, training, research, and private practice for over 22 years.

Carol M. Mantooth, MS, is the Director of Psychoeducational and Case Worker Services at the Andrews Center, a community mental health agency in Tyler, TX. She has been employed in various clinical capacities for Andrews Center for seven years. She is a former Director of Client Services at the East Texas Crisis Center where much of this treatment program was developed. She has also been employed by Tyler Junior College as a Psychology Instructor. She has a Master of Science degree in Psychology from the University of Texas at Tyler. She assisted in developing the couple counseling program at the Crisis Center, and she helped develop and implement the counseling program for couples in groups, for battered and formerly battered women in groups, and for batterers in groups.

WORKBOOK
to Accompany

ENDING
SPOUSE / PARTNER ABUSE

A Psychoeducational
Approach for Individuals
and Couples

Robert Geffner
with Carol Mantooth

 Springer Publishing Company
New York

Springer Publishing Company, Inc.
536 Broadway
New York, NY 10012-3955

Acquisitions Editor: Bill Tucker
Production Editor: Pamela Lankas
Cover design by James Scotto-Lavino

01 02 03 04 / 5 4 3

ISBN   0-8261-1272-2

Printed in the United States of America

Contents

I Forms and Questionnaires

Treatment Program Handouts

II Foundations and Brief Interventions

III   Communicating and Expressing Feelings

IV   Self-Management and Assertiveness

V Intimacy Issues and Relapse Prevention

I

Forms and Questionnaires

Demographic Data Sheet

Name of Client (Last, First, Middle)   Home phone   Work phone

Address (Street & No., City, Zip)

M S D W Sep

Marital status   Referred by

M F

Sex   Birthdate   Age   Education (Highest Completed)

Employed? Yes   No   By whom:_____ SS# _____

Where:_____ In what capacity:_____

Previous treatment? Yes   No   When: _____

   By whom: _____

HOUSEHOLD COMPOSITION

Number in household _____

Name	Age	Relationship

Relative/Contact person: _____
Relationship: _____
Address: _____
Home Phone: _____ Business Phone:_____

Family income per year:
_____ None   _____ $15,001 to $20,000
_____ $5,000 or less   _____ $20,000 to $25,000
_____ $5,001 to $10,000   _____ $25,001 or more
_____ $10,001 to $15,000   _____ Don't know

Presenting problem: _____

_____

Client Social History

Date _____   Client number_____

Client name _____

GENERAL INFORMATION

Name _____   SS# _____
Address _____
Home phone _____   Business phone _____
Age _____ Date of birth _____ Sex _____ Ethnic origin _____
Employed? Yes   No   Where _____
Marital status _____   Years married _____
Spouse's name _____   Age _____
Spouse employed?   Yes   No   Where _____
Number of children _____   Sex and age _____
Number of marriages _____   Duration of each _____
Education _____   Religious preference _____
Spouse's education _____   Spouse's religion _____
Military _____   Spouse's military _____

HOUSEHOLD COMPOSITION

Number in household _____
Name   Age   Relationship

_____
_____
_____
_____
_____

Relative/Contact person: _____
Relationship: _____
Address: _____
Home Phone: _____   Business Phone:_____

Referred by:

What are your specific needs?

Client Social History *(Continued)*

Client name: _____

CHILDHOOD: BIRTH TO AGE 12

Date of birth: _____ Place of birth: _____

Mother's condition during pregnancy: _____

Complications during delivery: _____

Developmental problems: _____

Check all of the following that applied during your childhood:

_____ Night terrors	_____ Bedwetting	_____ Sleepwalking
_____ Thumbsucking	_____ Nailbiting	_____ Stammering
_____ Fears	_____ Happy childhood	_____ Unhappy childhood
_____ Other		

Illnesses during childhood (age): _____

Surgery during childhood (age): _____

Accidents during childhood (age): _____

Fears during childhood: _____

Relationships with teachers: _____

Relationships with peers: _____

Relationships with parents: _____

Relationships with siblings: _____

Parent's religious preference: _____

Was your mother physically abused by your father? _____

Were you physically abused (by whom)? _____

Were you sexually abused (by whom)? _____

Feelings about school, problems, grades: _____

Problems with legal authorities (reason): _____

Counseling during childhood (by whom, what reason, how long?):

_____

_____

Were you treated in a mental hospital during childhood (where, age, what reason, how long)?

_____

_____

Client Social History *(Continued)*

Client name: _____

Problems during childhood with drugs/alcohol (to what extent):

_____

_____

Did you attempt suicide during childhood (when, what method did you use, for what reason)?

_____

Describe yourself as a child:

Check all of the following that you feel applied to you sometime as a child:

_____	Loss of self-esteem	_____	Personal guilt or shame
_____	Nervous symptoms (such as nailbiting)	_____	Feeling of maturity/responsibility inappropriate for age
_____	Sleep problems (including nightmares)		
_____	Self-damaging, self-destructive behavior	_____	Withdrawal from normal childhood activities
_____	Truancy and/or delinquency		
_____	Depression	_____	Eating disorders (overeating, fear of being overweight, overweight, underweight)
_____	Sudden change in school performance		
_____	Difficulty with social relationships		
_____	Running away from home	_____	Homicidal ideas (wanting to kill someone)
_____	Preoccupation with sexual matters		
_____	Sexual involvement before age 13	_____	Pregnancy
_____	Desire to have sexual involvement with same-sex partner	_____	Sexual abuse of younger children
		_____	The favored child in the family
_____	Isolated from friends	_____	Bedwetting
_____	Drug/alcohol use		

ADOLESCENCE: AGE 12–18

Where did you live as an teenager? _____

Illnesses during teenage years (age): _____

Surgery during teenage years (age): _____

Accidents during teenage years (age): _____

Fears during adolescence: _____

Relationships with teachers: _____

Relationships with peers: _____

Relationships with parents: _____

Relationships with siblings: _____

Client Social History *(Continued)*

Client name: _____

Was your mother physically abused by your father? _____

Were you physically abused (by whom)? _____

Were you sexually abused (by whom)? _____

Feelings about school, problems, grades: _____

Problems with legal authorities (for what reason): _____

Problems with drugs or alcohol (to what extent): _____

Counseling during teenage years (by whom, what reason, how long)?

_____

Were you treated in a mental hospital during teenage years (where, what age, what reason, how long)? _____

Did you attempt suicide during teenage years (when, what method, what reason)?

_____

At what age did you start dating? _____

Were you sexually active during teenage years (what age)? _____

At what age did you leave home? _____

Describe yourself as an adolescent:

ADULTHOOD: AGE 18 AND OVER

Number of brothers and sisters and their ages: _____

What is your birth order? _____

Are parents living?_____

Parents' education:_____

Parents' occupations: _____

Relationship with parents during adult years: _____

Relationship with children: _____

Relationship with spouse:_____

Age at each marriage: _____

Have you been sexually abused during your adulthood (by whom)?

_____

Have you been physically abused during your adulthood (by whom)?

_____

Client Social History *(Continued)*

Client name: _____

Problems with drugs/alcohol: _____

Problems with legal authorities (for what reason): _____

Counseling during adult years (by whom, what reason, how long?):

_____

Have you been treated in a mental hospital during the adult years (when, where, for what reason, how long)? _____

Have you attempted suicide during your adult years (when, what method, what reason)?

_____

Illnesses during adult years (age): _____

Accidents during adult years (age): _____

Surgery during adult years (age): _____

Describe the present problem and anything that relates to it. Please give details: _____

_____

_____

Describe your present job situation, number of jobs held in the past year, reasons for change:

_____

_____

Describe your present social involvement, and membership in any organizations: _____

_____

_____

Describe your present relationship with your family: _____

_____

_____

Describe how you spend your leisure time; what type activities do you find pleasurable:

_____

_____

Describe your present health, illnesses, medications: _____

_____

Describe how you handle stress: _____

_____

Client Social History *(Continued)*

Client name: _____

PRESENT

Please check any of the following that apply to you:

_____ Low self-esteem
_____ Sense of helplessness (feeling there is no solution)
_____ Prolonged physical symptoms/problems
_____ Eating disturbances (overeating, overweight, underweight, fear of being overweight)
_____ Frequent depression
_____ Hurting or desire to hurt yourself
_____ Lack of self-identity (difficulty describing who you are)
_____ Thoughts of suicide
_____ Passivity (not saying how you feel or what you want)
_____ Anger
_____ Aggression
_____ Guilt
_____ Clinically diagnosed psychological problems
_____ Conflict with partner
_____ Fear of partner
_____ Conflict with parents or in-laws
_____ Difficulty establishing and/or maintaining close friends
_____ Avoiding sexual involvement
_____ Unsatisfactory sexual relationship
_____ Sexual problems
_____ Thoughts of harming your own or other's children
_____ Other:

Confidentiality Statement

We place a high value on the confidentiality of the information that our clients share with us. This sheet was prepared to clarify our legal and ethical responsibilities regarding this important issue.

Personal information that you share with us may be entered into your records in written form. However, an effort is generally made to avoid entry of information that may be especially sensitive or embarrassing. The only individuals with access to our files are staff members who are either directly involved in providing services to you or those performing related clerical tasks. All of these persons are aware of the strict confidential nature of the information in the records. Persons from outside our office are not allowed access to our files without a court order or your written permission.

RELEASE OF INFORMATION TO OTHERS

If for some reason there is a need to share information in your record with someone not employed here (for example, your physician or another therapist), you will first be consulted and asked to sign a form authorizing transfer of the information. Because of the sensitive nature of the information contained in some records, you may wish to discuss the release of this material and related implications very carefully before you sign. The form will specify the information that you give us permission to release to the other party and will specify the time period during which the information may be released. You can revoke your permission at any time by simply giving us written notice.

EXCEPTIONS TO CONFIDENTIALITY

There are several important instances when confidential information may be released to others. First, if you have been referred to this agency by the court ("court ordered"), you can assume the court will wish to receive some type of report or evaluation. You should discuss with us exactly what information we would include in such a report to the court *before* you disclose any confidential material. In such instances, you have a right to tell us only what you want us to know.

Second, if you threaten to harm either yourself or someone else and we believe your threat to be serious, we are obligated under the law to take whatever actions seem necessary to protect you or others from harm. This may include divulging confidential information to others, and would only be done under unusual circumstances, when someone's life appears to be in danger.

Finally, if we have reason to believe that you are abusing or neglecting your children, we are obligated by law to report this to the appropriate state agency. The law is designed to protect children from harm and the obligations to report suspected abuse or neglect are clear in this regard.

In summary, we make every reasonable effort to safeguard the personal information that you may share with us. There are, however, certain instances when we may be obligated under the law to release such information to others. If you have any questions about confidentiality, please discuss them with us.

Confidentiality Release

(For staff) Explain the following areas of the Confidentiality Statement to each client. Give each client a copy of the Confidentiality Statement. Have each client sign this form.

   I. Confidentiality Statement

  II. Release of information to others

 III. Exceptions to confidentiality
       A. Court referrals
       B. Threats to harm yourself or others
       C. Abusing or neglecting your children
       D. Records subpoenaed

The Confidentiality Statement has been explained to me and I have received a copy. I have read and understand the Confidentiality Statement and agree to it.

_____   _____
             Client   Witness

                      _____
                                  Date

Client Consent Form

I, the undersigned, authorize _____ to:

Yes   No—Counsel me and enter me into treatment

Yes   No—Test and conduct assessment

Yes   No—Audio/Videotape (for staff supervision or to show to me at a later date)

Yes   No—Use basic information for research purposes

Yes   No—Other—Specify (and initial):_____

and release the above agency and staff thereof from liability.

_____

Client Signature

_____

Staff Signature

_____

Date

Consent for Follow-Up

Name_____   Client number _____

Address_____   Termination date _____

_____   Counselor _____

Home phone _____   Business phone _____

Date for follow-up after treatment concludes   Date follow-up completed

   1 month:_____   1 month: _____

   3 month:_____   3 month: _____

   6 month:_____   6 month: _____

   1 year:_____   1 year: _____

   2 years: _____   2 years: _____

May we contact you by mail? Yes   No
May we contact you by phone? Yes   No

How could we contact you if you are no longer at this address or telephone number?

_____

_____

Please contact us if your address or telephone number should change.

_____   _____
             Client   Staff

            _____
                 Date

Precounseling Questionnaire

Name _____   Client number_____

Classification_____   Date _____

1. How long has the violence been occurring before entering counseling? _____

2. What types of violence have occurred?

   Pushing/Shoving _____   Hair pulling _____
   Physical restraint _____   Cuts _____
   Slapping _____   Use of weapon or object _____
   Hitting _____   Threats to use a weapon _____
   Choking _____   Involuntary sex _____
   Punching _____   Verbal abuse _____
   Kicking_____   Burns _____
   Other: _____

3. How often has the violence occurred?

   Once _____   Once a week _____
   Once a month _____   2–3 times a week _____
   2–3 times a month _____   Daily _____
   Other: _____

4. Have you ever left home after a violent incident?   Yes   No

5. If yes, where did you go?

   To friend _____   For a walk _____
   To family _____   For a drive _____
   To shelter _____   To a club _____
   To motel _____   Other: _____

6. When was the last violent incident? _____

7. What do you think started the last abusive incident?

   Alcohol use _____   Conflicts about children_____
   Drug use _____   Conflicts about/with in-laws
   Unemployment _____   or other family members _____
   Job pressures _____   Jealousy _____
   Sexual demands _____   Financial/money pressures _____

   Physical aggression by partner (Describe): _____

   Other: _____

Precounseling Questionnaire *(Continued)*

8. What happened after the incident?

   Arguments _____   Police were called _____
   Calm discussion _____   Charges were filed_____
   I called other family member _____   Called agency for advice _____
   Spouse called other family member _____   I left the house/apt _____
   Spouse left the house/apt _____   Other (Specify): _____

9. Was there violence or abuse directed toward your children?   Yes   No

10. Was this violence or abuse: Physical _____   Verbal _____   Sexual _____

11. Under what conditions did you enter counseling?

    Voluntary, through self-referral_____
    Voluntary, through other agency _____
    Through court diversion, preplea _____
    Through court diversion, postplea _____
    Joint agreement between partner and self _____
    Other: _____

12. What issues would you like to see addressed in counseling sessions?

    Anger management _____   Exploration of gender roles _____
    Assertiveness training _____   Communication skill training _____
    Stress management _____   Self-esteem enhancement _____
    Parenting skills _____   Relationship enhancement _____
    Money management _____   Personality assessment_____
    Building social support   Drug/alcohol intervention
       systems _____   or treatment _____
    Emotional expression training _____   Emotional awareness training _____
    Support outside sessions (e.g.,   Problem-solving skill training _____
       hotline, access to program   Other: _____
       personnel, etc.)

Nonsuicide and No-Harm Contract

Name: _____ DOB: _____ Date: _____

I, _____ , agree not to do anything that might hurt

myself or anyone else before my next appointment on _____ with

my therapist(s) _____.

In addition, I agree that I will contact and talk to my therapist or the counselor on call by

telephoning the office/agency number,_____ , if I feel like hurting

myself or others. In case I cannot reach my therapist, I will call the emergency hotline of the

local crisis center at _____ for help.

Client: _____ Date: _____
                        Signature

Witness: _____
                        Signature

Nonviolence Contract

SELF-VIOLENCE

1. Have you ever thought about attempting suicide?   Yes   No

2. Have you ever attempted suicide?   Yes   No

3. If yes, how many times and when (approximately)?

   _____

4. What method did you use?

   _____

5. Have you thought of harming yourself recently?   Yes   No

SPOUSE/PARTNER VIOLENCE

1. Have you ever thought about being physically abusive toward your spouse/partner?
       Yes   No

2. Have you been abusive to your spouse/partner?   Yes   No

3. If yes, how many times and when (approximately)?

   _____

4. What form of abuse have you used? _____

5. Have you recently thought of harming your spouse/partner?   Yes   No

I will not attempt to harm myself or anyone else in any way.

Also, I will inform a member of the staff immediately if I think about or feel that I am about to harm myself or anyone else.

Client _____   Staff _____

Date _____

Aggressive Behavior Inventory

Client name: _____   Date: _____

Please list the approximate number of times you have been involved in the events listed below for each period of time indicated.

Happened to Me	Past week	One month	Two months	Three months	Past year
Pinching	_____	_____	_____	_____	_____
Slapping	_____	_____	_____	_____	_____
Grabbing	_____	_____	_____	_____	_____
Kicking	_____	_____	_____	_____	_____
Punching	_____	_____	_____	_____	_____
Hair pulling	_____	_____	_____	_____	_____
Throwing things	_____	_____	_____	_____	_____
Throwing partner or shoving	_____	_____	_____	_____	_____
Hitting with physical object	_____	_____	_____	_____	_____
Choking	_____	_____	_____	_____	_____
Threat of or use of weapon	_____	_____	_____	_____	_____
Burning	_____	_____	_____	_____	_____
Sexual abuse	_____	_____	_____	_____	_____
Destruction of property	_____	_____	_____	_____	_____
Verbal abuse	_____	_____	_____	_____	_____
Emotional abuse	_____	_____	_____	_____	_____

I Did to Partner	Past week	One month	Two months	Three months	Past year
Pinching	_____	_____	_____	_____	_____
Slapping	_____	_____	_____	_____	_____
Grabbing	_____	_____	_____	_____	_____
Kicking	_____	_____	_____	_____	_____
Punching	_____	_____	_____	_____	_____
Hair pulling	_____	_____	_____	_____	_____
Throwing things	_____	_____	_____	_____	_____
Throwing partner or shoving	_____	_____	_____	_____	_____
Hitting with physical object	_____	_____	_____	_____	_____
Choking	_____	_____	_____	_____	_____
Threat of or use of weapon	_____	_____	_____	_____	_____
Burning	_____	_____	_____	_____	_____
Sexual abuse	_____	_____	_____	_____	_____
Destruction of property	_____	_____	_____	_____	_____
Verbal abuse	_____	_____	_____	_____	_____
Emotional abuse	_____	_____	_____	_____	_____

Progress Evaluation Form

Client's name: _____

Group leader (Initials):_____ Date:_____ Session #: (circle one) 6 12 18 24

INSTRUCTIONS

Please rate the group member named above on each of the listed criteria. Use the 0 to 5 rating scale listed below, based on your impressions and observations. Obtain ratings from the client's partner, if possible, and also list below.

5 = occurs very often; 4 = often; 3 = occurs sometimes; 2 = not often;
1 = occurs rarely; 0 = unknown

_____ **Attendance:** Arrives at group session on time; attends regularly; contacts program in advance about absence; has legitimate excuse for absences.

_____ **Nonviolence:** Has not recently physically abused partner, children, or others; no apparent threats, intimidation, or manipulation.

_____ **Sobriety:** Attends meeting sober; no apparent abuse of alcohol or drugs during week; complying to ordered or referred drug and alcohol treatment.

_____ **Acceptance of responsibility:** Admits that violence and/or abuse occurred; not minimizing, blaming, or excusing problems; accepts responsibility for abuse, and contribution to problems.

_____ **Using techniques:** Takes steps to avoid abusiveness; refers to time-outs, self-talk, conflict-resolution skills, etc.; does homework assignments and follows recommendations.

_____ **Help-seeking:** Seeks information about alternatives; discusses options with others in the group; calls other participants for help; open to referrals and future support.

_____ **Actively engaged:** Attentive body language and nonverbal response; maintains eye contact; speaks with feeling; follows topic of discussion in comments; lets others speak; asks questions of others without interrogating; acknowledges others' contributions; participates.

_____ **Self-disclosure:** Reveals struggles, feelings, fears, and self-doubts; not withholding or evading issues; not sarcastic or defensive.

_____ **Sensitive language:** Respectful of partner and women in general; nonsexist language and no pejorative slang; checks others who use sexist language.

_____ **Empathy and insight:** Has insight concerning the abusiveness, its effects on the partner, and its dangerousness; understands the fears and trauma the abuse causes; realizes the negative impact of using power and controlling behaviors in relationships.

COMMENTS

Adapted from E. Gondolf, R. Foster, P. Burchfield, & D. Novosel (1995).

TREATMENT PROGRAM HANDOUTS

II

Foundations and
Brief Interventions

Weekly Behavior Inventory

Handout

Client name: _____   Date: _____

Please list the approximate number of times you have been involved in the events listed below during the last week. If you were the one slapped, etc., put the number of times. If you did the slapping, etc., put the number of times.

HAPPENED TO ME

Pinching   _____
Slapping   _____
Grabbing   _____
Kicking   _____
Punching   _____
Hair pulling   _____
Throwing things   _____
Throwing mate or shoving   _____
Hitting with physical object   _____
Choking   _____
Threat of or use of weapon   _____
Burning   _____
Sexual abuse   _____
Destruction of property   _____
Verbal abuse   _____
Emotional abuse   _____

HAPPENED TO CHILDREN

Pinching   _____
Slapping   _____
Grabbing   _____
Hair pulling   _____
Kicking   _____
Punching   _____
Throwing child   _____
Hitting with physical object   _____
Scarring child   _____
Use of weapon   _____
Threat of use of weapon   _____
Burning   _____
Sexual abuse   _____
Verbal abuse   _____
Emotional abuse   _____

I DID TO PARTNER

Pinching   _____
Slapping   _____
Grabbing   _____
Kicking   _____
Punching   _____
Hair pulling   _____
Throwing things   _____
Throwing mate or shoving   _____
Hitting with physical object   _____
Choking   _____
Threat of or use of weapon   _____
Burning   _____
Sexual abuse   _____
Destruction of property   _____
Verbal abuse   _____
Emotional abuse   _____
Acted assertively   _____
Communicated effectively   _____
Used time-out   _____
Controlled angry behavior   _____

I DID TO CHILDREN

Pinching   _____
Slapping   _____
Grabbing   _____
Hair pulling   _____
Kicking   _____
Punching   _____
Throwing child   _____
Hitting with physical object   _____
Scarring child   _____
Use of weapon   _____
Threat of use of weapon   _____
Burning   _____
Sexual abuse   _____
Verbal abuse   _____
Emotional abuse   _____
Acted assertively   _____
Communicated effectively   _____
Used time-out   _____
Controlled angry behavior   _____
Spent quality time   _____

I DID HOMEWORK   _____

I DON'T FEEL SAFE
TALKING IN GROUP   _____

Group Orientation

Handout

Welcome to group therapy. The following is a list of answers to frequently asked questions about the groups. Please read this information carefully.

1. Why were you referred?

   You were referred to this program because of a report that indicated that you were involved in an incident of family violence. The fact that you have been referred to one of our groups indicates that your problem is treatable. If your partner is also in treatment with you, it usually means she made the decision to stay in the relationship and to take part in the program.

2. How often do the groups meet?

   Each group meets for 1½–2 hours, once a week for 26 weeks, followed by 6 monthly meetings.

3. What happens in the group?

   Treatment is divided into four modules. Each module is designed to focus on a particular aspect of ending family violence and on improving important skills. Groups provide an atmosphere in which members can discuss the problems they have encountered, the feelings that have led to the abusive behavior, and the impact abuse has had on the relationship. New ways of communicating, handling stress, and resolving conflicts are strongly emphasized.

4. Is this a class or group therapy?

   Although many of the group sessions may involve teaching of specific skills, such as stress management and improved communication, the groups are considered to be group therapy. This means that there is a strong emphasis placed on self-examination, discussion of feelings, and support for other group members. Most people benefit from the group process based on how committed they are to engage in these tasks.

5. Do I have to come every week?

   Group members have agreed or have been required to attend. The attendance of wives/partners is voluntary. It is not the responsibility of male members to persuade their partners to come to group. Nor is it acceptable for male members to discourage their partners from attending group. Interference of this kind is grounds for dismissal from treatment with associated consequences. In order for you to benefit from the program, attendance must become a priority. As you become more involved in the group, you will probably find that you are motivated to attend, not only for your own benefit, but also to support your fellow group members. You should attend each session even if your spouse/partner is unable to attend.

6. What about absences?

   The staff recognizes that commitments may require you to miss a group meeting. If you are unable to attend a group session for such a reason, contact the program staff ahead of time at the phone number given. Documentation of all excused absences is required, and the homework or other assignments must be completed before the next session. Undocumented absences and those that occur without notification will be considered unexcused.

   You will be required to attend weekly meetings for 6 months. No more than two excused absences can be allowed in any module. If more absences occur, then you will be required to begin the module again; if absences become a pattern, then you will be subject to possible probation/termination from the program.

Group Orientation *(Continued)*

Handout

Unexcused absences, that is, those that occur not as a result of documented prior commitments that cannot be changed and/or illness, indicate a lack of interest or commitment to the decision to change your situation. One unexcused absence will result in the authorities (if relevant) being notified of your failure to attend group. Two unexcused absences will result in your being placed on probation with notification to relevant authorities. Any additional unexcused absences may result in termination from the program. Late arrivals to the start of group will be considered an unexcused absence.

You will also be required to attend six monthly meetings after the 6 months of weekly meetings have been completed. These are large-group meetings that provide follow-up, networking with others, and the opportunity to address issues on how to use the skills you have learned. Your case will be reviewed for closure after the completion of six monthly meetings. Wives/partners are encouraged to attend even when their partners are absent.

7. Who leads the groups?

All of the group leaders are mental health professionals who have had extensive training in the particular treatment you will receive. Groups may be co-led by both a female and male therapist.

8. Are there additional expectations for successful participation other than group attendance?

Most sessions have homework assignments that you will be expected to complete and bring to the next group meeting. The therapists will review the homework assignment with you at the end of each group meeting so you will know what is expected for the next session. Therapists will discuss the completed homework at the beginning of each group meeting. Failure to complete homework on three occasions will be considered the equivalent of one unexcused absence.

You will be given a three-ring binder at the first group meeting. You are expected to bring your binder to each group meeting.

9. What about confidentiality? Can what I say in the group be used against me?

Because this treatment uses a "team" approach among therapists you can assume that what you say in the group may be discussed with staff members. In order to effectively prepare progress notes regarding your treatment, a case manager may review your progress with the group leaders. Only information that is directly related to your treatment goals is included in these reports. Most of the personal issues and feelings discussed in the group sessions remain confidential.

In certain situations, the group leaders are obligated to report information that is revealed in the group. These reportable situations include serious threats of hurting or killing someone else, serious threats of hurting or killing yourself, reports of child abuse, or current use of illegal drugs.

10. What about new incidents of abuse?

a. If the new incident is of a formal nature (i.e., comes from the Court, the police, the military, a medical treatment facility, etc.), the case will be referred to relevant staff for review and disposition. If the incident is substantiated, the following options exist:

- Terminate services and return the case to relevant authorities, if appropriate.

Group Orientation (*Continued*)

Handout

- Place the group member on probation with the provision that a new incident of violence will be cause for the termination of treatment. Services will continue.
- Amend the treatment plan.

b. If information regarding an incident of violence surfaces as a result of treatment (i.e., the regular surveys used in treatment, interaction with therapists and case managers), case managers and therapists will make clinical judgments regarding the continuation of services and/or referral of your case to relevant authorities for disposition. All incidents of serious abuse will be reported, but continuation of the treatment program will be made on a case-by-case basis.

ADDITIONAL INFORMATION AND OTHER GROUP RULES

1. Groups begin at the designated time. Group members are required to be at the center 10 minutes before the group's start time in order to fill out a questionnaire entitled "Weekly Behavior Inventory." Groups will not begin until everyone completes the questionnaire. Failure to complete the questionnaire will result in an unexcused absence for the group member.

2. Alcohol must not be used the day of group.

3. Group members will not threaten nor intimidate any group members or therapists at any time. Therapists and clients will ensure the safety of all group members.

4. When the treatment includes couples, each individual will return home separately after the group whenever possible or when directed by the group therapists. Carpooling for members of the same gender is encouraged.

5. If couples separate or divorce after group treatment has started, they can still decide to continue treatment, either in the same group or in different groups. Those group members who are required to remain in treatment will do so, either in the same group or in another one until completion of the program.

6. Group sessions may be audio or videotaped to ensure that group therapists are delivering treatment services in the appropriate order and manner. The focus is on the therapists, not the participants. The tapes will be used for *no other purpose*. The only people with access to the audiotapes are those who oversee the work of the therapists.

7. The leaders of the groups will evaluate your progress every 6–8 weeks. These evaluations will be used to assess your progress.

8. You will be asked to evaluate your progress every 6–8 weeks. These evaluations will also be used to assess your progress.

9. You will be asked to evaluate your group leaders every 6–8 weeks. These evaluations will be used to evaluate the work the group leaders are doing.

I have read the above information and agree to the conditions of treatment.

_____   _____
Group Member's Signature   Witness Signature

_____
Date

Counseling and Support Group Assumptions and Rules

Handout

Some assumptions have been made in putting this group together.

THESE ASSUMPTIONS ARE

1. Each of us is in this group because we have had a similar experience.
2. Each person can best define how he or she feels about his or her situation or experiences. No assumptions will be made about how anyone "should" or "should not" feel.
3. Each person can best decide what, if anything, he or she wants to do about his or her experiences and decide what changes he or she may want to make in his or her life. No assumptions will be made about how anyone "should" or "should not" act. It is made clear, however, that violent and abusive acts are to be eliminated, and that is one of the main reasons we are here.
4. Each person's experiences are valid and important. They cannot be judged as better or worse than anyone else's experiences.
5. Each of us has inner strengths.
6. This group is meant to be a sharing experience. It is not intended for us as facilitators just to talk to you, but for you to talk to each other. We can support each other and learn from each other.

RULES

1. Once a person decides to enter the group, it should be viewed as a commitment. It is expected that you will come every week except for emergencies. Your presence is needed for continuity. You are truly missed when you are absent. Call if you cannot attend a meeting. The group members need you even when you do not need them.
2. Membership in the group will be limited. When that limit is reached, other people will be put on a waiting list. They will enter the next group formed.
3. Groups will run for a period of 26 sessions, with 6 monthly follow-up sessions.
4. Everything said in the group is confidential. Nothing said by anyone should be used in conversations outside the group. No information heard in group about other members will be discussed with or mentioned to anyone who is not a group member.
5. Each person is his or her own best judge of what he or she feels is okay to talk about in the group meetings. Each is responsible for setting his or her own limits.

The Nine Basic Rules

Handout

1. We are all 100% responsible for our behavior.

2. Violence is not an acceptable solution to problems.

3. We do not have control over any other person, but we can control ourselves.

4. When communicating with someone else, we need to express our feelings directly rather than blaming or threatening the other person.

5. Increased awareness of self-talk, physical cues, and emotions is essential for progress and improvement.

6. We can always take a *"time-out"* before reacting.

7. We can't do anything about the past, but we can change the future.

8. Although there are differences between men and women, our needs and rights are fundamentally alike.

9. Counselors and case managers cannot make people change—they can only set the stage for change to occur.

House of Abuse

Handout

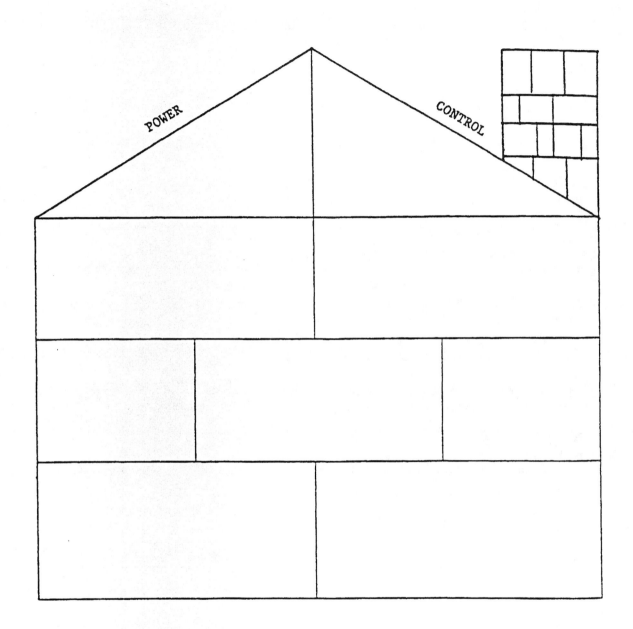

Developed by: Michael F. McGrane, Wilder Foundation, Community Assistance Program, 650 Marshall Avenue, St. Paul, MN 55104.

Emotional/Psychological Abuse

Handout

Psychological/emotional abuse always accompanies and, in many cases, precedes physical battering. Like hitting, targeted and repeated emotional abuse can have severe effects on the victim's sense of self and reality. Use of this list may help answer the perennial question, "Why do battered women stay?"

BRAINWASHING

- Jokes about habits/faults
- Insults
- Ignoring feelings
- Withholding approval as punishment
- Yelling
- Name calling
- Repeated insults/targeted insults
- Repeated humiliation (public)
- Repeated humiliation (private)
- Labeling as "crazy," "bitch," whore," "animal,"and so on
- Threatens violence/retaliation
- Puts down abilities as parent, worker, and lover
- Demands all of the attention (resents children)
- Tells about affairs
- Threatens with abusing children or getting custody
- Offers to stay because he/she "needs" the partner and can't make it alone

POSSIBLE CONSEQUENCES TO VICTIM

- Powerlessness/learned helplessness
- Unpredictable consequences of actions
- Questions sense of reality
- Nervous breakdown, depression
- Dependency
- Emotional instability
- Suicide or attempts

Adapted from Wexler (1990).

© 1999 Springer Publishing Company.

Sexual Abuse and Violence

Handout

This is the most difficult aspect of family abuse to identify and discuss, whether in a group or individually. Sexual abuse in the home is, however, more common than many would like to believe. Raising awareness of the possibility of child sexual abuse and giving you permission to articulate your own sexual victimization as a child or in the adult relationship, if these occurred, are expected outcomes of this exercise.

INCEST:
Many women and men were sexually abused in childhood, mostly by family members.

RAPE:
This occurs in and outside of marriage.

Sexual abuse includes the following:

- Jokes about women said in their presence.
- Sexual "put-down" jokes.
- Women/men seen as a sex object (leering).
- Minimizing feelings and needs regarding sex.
- Criticizing sexual "performance."
- Sexual labels: "whore" may alternate with "frigid."
- Unwanted touch.
- Uncomfortable touch (or forced to touch/made to watch others).
- Withholding sex and affection.
- Always wanting sex.
- Demanding sex with threats.
- Forced to strip—humiliation (maybe in front of kids).
- Promiscuity with others.
- Forced to watch.
- Jealousy—may be extreme.
- Forced sex with him or others.
- Forced uncomfortable sex.
- Forced sex after beatings.
- Sex for the purpose of hurting (use of objects/weapons).
- Sexual torture.
- Murder.

Adapted from Wexler (1990).

Weekly Behavior Inventory

Client name: _____   Date: _____

Please list the approximate number of times you have been involved in the events listed below during the last week. If you were the one slapped, etc., put the number of times. If you did the slapping, etc., put the number of times.

HAPPENED TO ME

Pinching ____
Slapping ____
Grabbing ____
Kicking ____
Punching ____
Hair pulling ____
Throwing things ____
Throwing mate or shoving ____
Hitting with physical object ____
Choking ____
Threat of or use of weapon ____
Burning ____
Sexual abuse ____
Destruction of property ____
Verbal abuse ____
Emotional abuse ____

HAPPENED TO CHILDREN

Pinching ____
Slapping ____
Grabbing ____
Hair pulling ____
Kicking ____
Punching ____
Throwing child ____
Hitting with physical object ____
Scarring child ____
Use of weapon ____
Threat of use of weapon ____
Burning ____
Sexual abuse ____
Verbal abuse ____
Emotional abuse ____

I DID TO PARTNER

Pinching ____
Slapping ____
Grabbing ____
Kicking ____
Punching ____
Hair pulling ____
Throwing things ____
Throwing mate or shoving ____
Hitting with physical object ____
Choking ____
Threat of or use of weapon ____
Burning ____
Sexual abuse ____
Destruction of property ____
Verbal abuse ____
Emotional abuse ____
Acted assertively ____
Communicated effectively ____
Used time-out ____
Controlled angry behavior ____

I DID TO CHILDREN

Pinching ____
Slapping ____
Grabbing ____
Hair pulling ____
Kicking ____
Punching ____
Throwing child ____
Hitting with physical object ____
Scarring child ____
Use of weapon ____
Threat of use of weapon ____
Burning ____
Sexual abuse ____
Verbal abuse ____
Emotional abuse ____
Acted assertively ____
Communicated effectively ____
Used time-out ____
Controlled angry behavior ____
Spent quality time ____

I DID HOMEWORK ____

I DON'T FEEL SAFE
TALKING IN GROUP ____

Safety-and-Control Plan

TIME-OUT PLAN

(If you need to leave, what will tell you that you need to go; what will you do to leave; or while leaving, where will you go; what will you do?)

"BUDDY'S" NUMBER:

(A good friend from group or otherwise.)

GROUP NUMBERS:

(Alternative phone numbers in case "buddy" is not home.)

PREVIOUS PLANS

(What have you done in the past to help yourself cool down or deal with anger in an appropriate way?)

PHYSICAL-EXERCISE PLAN

(How can you work off energy or anxiety in a nondestructive way, sport, or other activity?)

STRESS-REDUCTION PLAN

(What do you enjoy doing, something that relaxes you and helps you think straight?)

Emergency: _____   Battered Women:_____

Crisis Line: _____   Child Abuse: _____

AA: _____   E. R.: _____

Taken from Wexler (1990).

© 1999 Springer Publishing Company.

Weekly Behavior Inventory

Handout

Client name: _____   Date: _____

Please list the approximate number of times you have been involved in the events listed below during the last week. If you were the one slapped, etc., put the number of times. If you did the slapping, etc., put the number of times.

HAPPENED TO ME

Pinching ____
Slapping ____
Grabbing ____
Kicking ____
Punching ____
Hair pulling ____
Throwing things ____
Throwing mate or shoving ____
Hitting with physical object ____
Choking ____
Threat of or use of weapon ____
Burning ____
Sexual abuse ____
Destruction of property ____
Verbal abuse ____
Emotional abuse ____

I DID TO PARTNER

Pinching ____
Slapping ____
Grabbing ____
Kicking ____
Punching ____
Hair pulling ____
Throwing things ____
Throwing mate or shoving ____
Hitting with physical object ____
Choking ____
Threat of or use of weapon ____
Burning ____
Sexual abuse ____
Destruction of property ____
Verbal abuse ____
Emotional abuse ____
Acted assertively ____
Communicated effectively ____
Used time-out ____
Controlled angry behavior ____

I DID HOMEWORK ____

HAPPENED TO CHILDREN

Pinching ____
Slapping ____
Grabbing ____
Hair pulling ____
Kicking ____
Punching ____
Throwing child ____
Hitting with physical object ____
Scarring child ____
Use of weapon ____
Threat of use of weapon ____
Burning ____
Sexual abuse ____
Verbal abuse ____
Emotional abuse ____

I DID TO CHILDREN

Pinching ____
Slapping ____
Grabbing ____
Hair pulling ____
Kicking ____
Punching ____
Throwing child ____
Hitting with physical object ____
Scarring child ____
Use of weapon ____
Threat of use of weapon ____
Burning ____
Sexual abuse ____
Verbal abuse ____
Emotional abuse ____
Acted assertively ____
Communicated effectively ____
Used time-out ____
Controlled angry behavior ____
Spent quality time ____

I DON'T FEEL SAFE
TALKING IN GROUP ____

Basic Anger Management— What About Anger?

Handout

WHAT IS ANGER?

- An emotion like love, fear or joy.
- A feeling. It affects the way you experience life.
- A communication. It sends information to others.
- A cause. It produces specific effects and results (Weisinger, 1985).

Anger tells us there is something wrong that needs changing. It is important to growth and adjustment to learn to feel and express a wide range of emotions. Anger is normal. Inappropriate behavior is not "normal," however. Inappropriate behavior is exhibited by physical violence, threats, verbally abusive comments, and sexual abuse.

ANGER TRIGGERS

- Frustration
- Extreme stress
- Feeling put down
- Fear of rejection
- Social learning experience
- Someone hurts you

THREE COMPONENTS OF ANGER

- Physiological—This is exemplified by body changes, such as sweating, increased heart rate, quickened breathing, trembling, brain-wave pattern changes, facial flushing.
- Feeling—Anger shows itself with changes in affect, tense, emotional, depressed thinking, "flight or fight" response.
- Expressive—Anger can be expressed through violent verbal outbursts, physical violence, threats of violence (slamming doors, etc.), or creative expression such as art, music, writing, sports, energized behaviors, and so on.

WHEN IS ANGER DYSFUNCTIONAL?

- When it is excessive, frequent, prolonged, or expressed inappropriately.

WHAT FACTORS INFLUENCE ANGER?

- Degree of arousal, awareness
- Past learning
- Past experience
- Present situation

Basic Anger Management— What About Anger? *(Continued)*

Handout

- Interpretation of the arousal
- Environment
- Temperament, personality
- Self-esteem

WHY DOESN'T EVERYONE EXPERIENCE THE SAME EMOTIONAL REACTIONS IN A SITUATION?

- Different past experiences
- Focus on different cues to explain the arousal
- Label feelings differently
- Different personalities

EFFECTS OF ANGER

- Positive— Can motivate and energize behavior
  Creative expressions, such as art, music, writing
- Negative—Physical problems, illness
  Mental and emotional problems
  Lowered self-esteem
  Work problems
  Relationship problems
  Behavioral problems, violence

HOW CAN YOU TELL WHEN YOUR SPOUSE IS GETTING ANGRY?

- Behavior—Slamming doors, stomping feet
- Verbal—Sarcastic tone, attitude, talking loudly, gruff, saying directly that he is angry
- Bodily cues—Face flushes, ears turn red, tense body posture, fists clinched

HOW DO YOU REACT TO YOUR SPOUSE'S ANGER?

- Get angry
- Ignore it
- Walk away
- Leave the house
- Withdraw in fear
- Other _____

Basic Anger Management— What About Anger? *(Continued)*

Handout

SOME WAYS TO DEAL WITH ANGER

- Be aware of your body's cues.
- Identify the source of the anger. Why are you angry?
- Deal with the situation or problem causing the anger.
- Talk to someone.
- Accept anger as normal; however, remember inappropriate behavior is not "normal."

There are many other ways of dealing with anger. Refer to the homework handout, other references, or recommended books.

Appropriate Alternatives to Violence

Handout

You Cannot Hurt Living Things or Any Property Not Expressly Obtained for That Reason. The Actions Must Not Intimidate Your Partner, Affect Your Partner's Property, or Scare Your Partner.

Alternatives to violence can be decided on jointly or suggested by counselors. The following is a list of ways to direct anger into harmless behavior.

Jogging or Walking Briskly—This is a benefit both for stress reduction and general health. When you feel good physically, you can confront stressful situations better. Also, the physical activity helps divert attention away from the stressful environment. A walk around the block is good if you cannot jog.

Physical Work or Exercise—Physical work and exercise can release energy while at the same time leading to a constructive accomplishment. The exercise can be at home or where you work.

Tearing Cardboard or Magazines—Any available scraps of cardboard or magazines are usable. You merely take the object and continue tearing until physically exhausted. This physical activity works off excessive anger.

Time-Out—This is getting off alone for awhile. You can listen to music, just sit quietly and daydream, or walk alone someplace where it is restful, such as a park, lake, woods, and so on. (Perhaps the couple can set a time limit for this.) You can also have a room at home where you can go to be away from everything for a while.

Deep Breathing—Just stop for a minute when you feel tension and take some deep breaths. This adds oxygen to the body, and helps you think more clearly, calm down, and change the focus from the situation. Also stretching or walking around while taking deep breaths can help.

Talking—Talking about the stressful situation to another person is helpful. Anyone who will take time to listen will be okay; the idea is to just talk about what is bothering you. Awareness of the physical symptoms prior to anger and then talking before "blowing up" will help reduce stress.

Relaxation Procedures—Tense and relax muscle groups. Refer to the relaxation session in the manual in Session 4.

Weekly Behavior Inventory

Handout

Client name: _____ Date: _____

Please list the approximate number of times you have been involved in the events listed below during the last week. If you were the one slapped, etc., put the number of times. If you did the slapping, etc., put the number of times.

HAPPENED TO ME

Pinching   ____
Slapping   ____
Grabbing   ____
Kicking   ____
Punching   ____
Hair pulling   ____
Throwing things   ____
Throwing mate or shoving   ____
Hitting with physical object   ____
Choking   ____
Threat of or use of weapon   ____
Burning   ____
Sexual abuse   ____
Destruction of property   ____
Verbal abuse   ____
Emotional abuse   ____

HAPPENED TO CHILDREN

Pinching   ____
Slapping   ____
Grabbing   ____
Hair pulling   ____
Kicking   ____
Punching   ____
Throwing child   ____
Hitting with physical object   ____
Scarring child   ____
Use of weapon   ____
Threat of use of weapon   ____
Burning   ____
Sexual abuse   ____
Verbal abuse   ____
Emotional abuse   ____

I DID TO PARTNER

Pinching   ____
Slapping   ____
Grabbing   ____
Kicking   ____
Punching   ____
Hair pulling   ____
Throwing things   ____
Throwing mate or shoving   ____
Hitting with physical object   ____
Choking   ____
Threat of or use of weapon   ____
Burning   ____
Sexual abuse   ____
Destruction of property   ____
Verbal abuse   ____
Emotional abuse   ____
Acted assertively   ____
Communicated effectively   ____
Used time-out   ____
Controlled angry behavior   ____

I DID HOMEWORK   ____

I DID TO CHILDREN

Pinching   ____
Slapping   ____
Grabbing   ____
Hair pulling   ____
Kicking   ____
Punching   ____
Throwing child   ____
Hitting with physical object   ____
Scarring child   ____
Use of weapon   ____
Threat of use of weapon   ____
Burning   ____
Sexual abuse   ____
Verbal abuse   ____
Emotional abuse   ____
Acted assertively   ____
Communicated effectively   ____
Used time-out   ____
Controlled angry behavior   ____
Spent quality time   ____

I DON'T FEEL SAFE TALKING IN GROUP   ____

Stress-Reduction Techniques

Handout

1. Learn to relax and enjoy some pleasant, fun things in life.

2. Get physical exercise on a regular basis.

3. Accept things and situations that cannot be changed.

4. Eat properly.

5. Set priorities in your life.

6. Learn to delegate.

7. Break the routine periodically. Do not get in a rut.

8. Use relaxation methods wherever you are. For example, use them while you are stopped at a red light.

9. Keep a diary for 2 weeks to note what upsets you. See if there is a pattern and what changes can be made.

10. Retreat from everyone for 15–30 minutes a day so you can relax and be alone.

11. Give yourself and others permission to feel their experiences.

12. Reward yourself when you handle a situation effectively and do not use violent methods.

13. Talk to your spouse or someone else about the stress you feel.

14. Learn to recognize your body's physiological response to stress.

15. Do not expect yourself or others to be perfect.

Methods of Relaxation

1. **Deep Breathing**   Take a deep breath and let it out very slowly. Try to take twice as long to exhale as to inhale. Breathe deep, down into your abdomen, not just your chest, then exhale very slowly. Do this for a few minutes several times a day.

2. **Meditation**   This can be used if you are already aware of this technique.

3. **Autogenic Exercise**   While in a relaxed and comfortable position, slowly say to yourself "warm and heavy." Repeat this to yourself over and over.

4. **Environment Awareness Exercise**   Choose a comfortable chair. As you are sitting in the chair, think about the chair and be aware of how it is supporting you. Let the chair be the support instead of your body doing the work.

5. **Deep-Muscle Relaxation**   While breathing deeply, tense and relax each muscle from head to toe. Focus on each muscle as you do this. Practice this at least twice a day.

6. **Mental Imagery**   Think of a very peaceful, soothing, and relaxing scene. You could picture a peaceful blue sky, a lovely green meadow, and so forth. While focusing on this, breathe slowly and naturally.

7. **Do Something for Someone Else**   Sign up for some volunteer work, do something for the family, or do something for a neighbor or elderly person.

8. **Personal Relaxation Program**   Usually, such a program would include three components: Progressive Muscle Relaxation, Breathing Exercises, and/or Mental Imagery. An example of such a program is:

   - Sit in a chair and relax your body (your arms and jaw should be "loose").
   - Close your eyes and erase all thoughts from your mind.
   - Create in your imagination a vivid, soothing mental scene . . . a peaceful sky, a green valley, ocean waves, and so forth.
   - Focus on breathing slowly and deeply . . . let your breath out slowly.
   - For additional relaxation, repeat a phrase or sound that you find soothing (such as the word "flower" or the number "one").
   - Repeat this exercise at least three times each day, whether or not you are tense, for about 30 to 50 seconds.
   - After 2 weeks, your body will be conditioned to relax whenever you do this exercise, and you will feel yourself calming down.

Weekly Behavior Inventory

Handout

Client name: _____ Date: _____

Please list the approximate number of times you have been involved in the events listed below during the last week. If you were the one slapped, etc., put the number of times. If you did the slapping, etc., put the number of times.

HAPPENED TO ME

Pinching   _____
Slapping   _____
Grabbing   _____
Kicking   _____
Punching   _____
Hair pulling   _____
Throwing things   _____
Throwing mate or shoving   _____
Hitting with physical object   _____
Choking   _____
Threat of or use of weapon   _____
Burning   _____
Sexual abuse   _____
Destruction of property   _____
Verbal abuse   _____
Emotional abuse   _____

HAPPENED TO CHILDREN

Pinching   _____
Slapping   _____
Grabbing   _____
Hair pulling   _____
Kicking   _____
Punching   _____
Throwing child   _____
Hitting with physical object   _____
Scarring child   _____
Use of weapon   _____
Threat of use of weapon   _____
Burning   _____
Sexual abuse   _____
Verbal abuse   _____
Emotional abuse   _____

I DID TO PARTNER

Pinching   _____
Slapping   _____
Grabbing   _____
Kicking   _____
Punching   _____
Hair pulling   _____
Throwing things   _____
Throwing mate or shoving   _____
Hitting with physical object   _____
Choking   _____
Threat of or use of weapon   _____
Burning   _____
Sexual abuse   _____
Destruction of property   _____
Verbal abuse   _____
Emotional abuse   _____
Acted assertively   _____
Communicated effectively   _____
Used time-out   _____
Controlled angry behavior   _____

I DID HOMEWORK   _____

I DID TO CHILDREN

Pinching   _____
Slapping   _____
Grabbing   _____
Hair pulling   _____
Kicking   _____
Punching   _____
Throwing child   _____
Hitting with physical object   _____
Scarring child   _____
Use of weapon   _____
Threat of use of weapon   _____
Burning   _____
Sexual abuse   _____
Verbal abuse   _____
Emotional abuse   _____
Acted assertively   _____
Communicated effectively   _____
Used time-out   _____
Controlled angry behavior   _____
Spent quality time   _____

I DON'T FEEL SAFE
TALKING IN GROUP   _____

Reducing Stress and Anger

Handout

You can reduce stress and anger with a technique called "desensitization." This helps you cope with situations that are threatening or frustrating to you. The key to desensitization is being able to relax while you imagine scenes that progressively become more stressful or anger provoking. As you learn to relax while imagining threatening or frustrating situations, you can transfer the results to life situations.

TWO PRINCIPLES OF SYSTEMATIC DESENSITIZATION

1. One emotion (relaxation) can be used to counteract another (anger).
2. A person can adjust to threatening and upsetting situations and have a minor emotional reaction.

STEPS IN USING AN ANGER LADDER (SYSTEMATIC DESENSITIZATION)

1. Take several days or more to learn to relax. This step is important because you learn that it is impossible to be physically relaxed and emotionally tense at the same time. There is a physiological link between your body and your mind. Choose a specific relaxation technique from Session 4, and practice it several times a day.

2. Make a list on the *Anger Ladder* of situations or experiences in which you have become angry.

3. Group all of the experiences or situations that bother you according to their common themes.

4. Put these situations in order, ranked from the lowest to highest levels in producing anger and anxiety. A high-level example might be that you get very angry if your spouse is late and has not called. This list is like a "ladder" of least disturbing, upsetting scenes that climbs to those that are most upsetting.

5. Start practicing the relaxation techniques in group. Visualize the scenes in your list, with the lowest first. As the anxiety builds, continue practicing the relaxation technique in group. Continue this process with each situation that produces anger. Go up your "ladder" gradually to the more upsetting scenes. Do not go higher until you are able to picture the scene while remaining calm. After you practice this in the group, continue imagining the lower level anxiety scenes on a daily basis. This process will take a few weeks overall.

ROLE PLAY

Example: A person you work with has a tendency to irritate you with his or her behavior. You have talked with this person, but he or she continues to irritate you. Shift into relaxation response so that his or her behavior does not bother you.

An Anger Ladder

Handout

An *Anger Ladder* is used to help you overcome the stress associated with anger. You can list five situations that produce varying levels of anger, and then rank them from least stressful to most stressful and anger provoking. You can also list and describe below, next to number 5, a situation that has made or would make you most angry. Next, list and describe a situation after number 1 below that has made or would make you the least angry. Then fill in situations for numbers 2–4 that produce increasing levels of anger, frustration, and anxiety. Your counselor or group leader will help you use these anger-producing scenes in combination with relaxation to help you overcome stress and better cope with anger.

1. Low Anger: _____
   _____
   _____
   _____
   _____

2. _____
   _____
   _____
   _____
   _____

3. _____
   _____
   _____
   _____
   _____

4. _____
   _____
   _____
   _____
   _____

5. Extreme Anger: _____
   _____
   _____
   _____

Before beginning to think about these situations, remember to review your relaxation techniques. Think about the first situation or least anger-producing situation in your life. This could consist of specific incidents with your spouse that triggered an angry reaction in yourself. As you are thinking about this situation and starting to feel your body react to the situation, begin applying the relaxation techniques that you have learned. You will notice yourself not reacting so strongly to the situation. Do this several times with each item on your list until you are comfortable thinking about these things, talking about them, and being in the situation face to face. This may take several sessions.

Cycle-of-Violence Behaviors

Handout

TENSION BUILDING

His Behavior

- Moody
- Nitpicks
- Isolates her
- Withdraws affection
- Puts her down
- Yells
- Drinks or takes drugs
- Threatens
- Destroys property
- Criticizes
- Acts sullen
- Crazy-making

Her Behavior

- Attempts to calm him
- Nurtures
- Silent/talkative
- Stays away from family, friends
- Keeps kids quiet
- Agrees
- Withdraws
- Tries to reason
- Cooks his favorite dinner
- Feels like always walking on eggshells

ACUTE EXPLOSION

His Behavior

- Humiliates
- Isolates her
- Abuses verbally
- Hits
- Chokes
- Uses weapons
- Beats
- Rapes
- Other abusive or violent behaviors

Her Behavior

- Protects herself anyway she can
- Police called by her, her kids, neighbors
- Tries to calm him
- Tries to reason
- Leaves
- Fights back

CALMING

His Behavior

- Shows remorse/begs forgiveness
- Promises to get counseling, go to church, AA
- Send flowers, bring presents
- Says, "I'll never do it again."
- Wants to make love
- Declares love
- Enlists family support
- Cries

Her Behavior

- Agrees to stay, returns, or takes him back
- Attempts to stop legal proceedings
- Sets up counseling appointment for him
- Feels happy, hopeful

Cycle-of-Violence Behaviors *(Continued)*

Denial works in each stage of the cycle to keep the cycle going (only by breaking through this denial can the cycle be broken):

TENSION BUILDING

His Behavior

- He denies by blaming the tension on her, work, the traffic, anything; by getting drunk or taking drugs; denies responsibility for his actions.

Her Behavior

- She denies that it's happening, excuses it to some outside stress (work, etc.); blames herself for his behavior, denies that the abuse will worsen.

EXPLOSION

His Behavior

- He blames it on her, stress, etc. ("She had it coming.")

Her Behavior

- She denies her injuries and minimizes them ("I bruise easily," didn't require police or medical help); blames it on drinking ("He didn't know what he was doing"); does not label it rape because it was her husband.

CALMING

His Behavior

- He believes it won't happen again.

Her Behavior

- She minimizes injuries ("It could have been worse"); believes this is the way it will stay, the man of her dreams, believes his promises.

Adapted from: Wexler and Saunders (1991).

The Cycle Theory of Violence

Handout

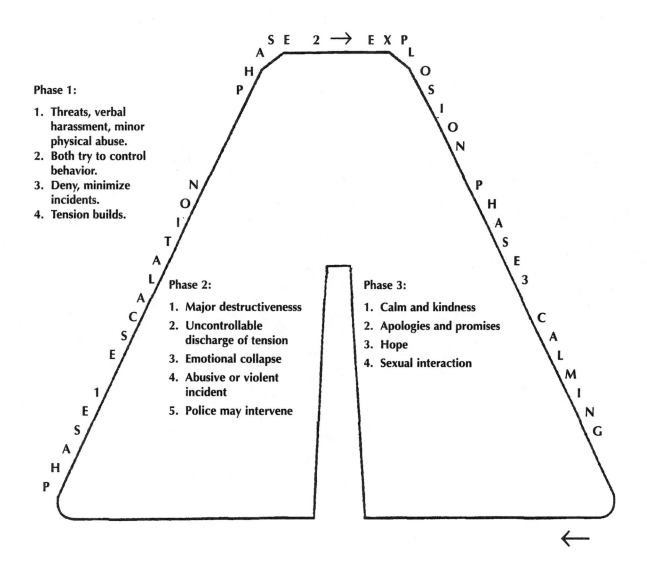

Phase 1:

1. Threats, verbal harassment, minor physical abuse.
2. Both try to control behavior.
3. Deny, minimize incidents.
4. Tension builds.

Phase 2:

1. Major destructivenesss
2. Uncontrollable discharge of tension
3. Emotional collapse
4. Abusive or violent incident
5. Police may intervene

Phase 3:

1. Calm and kindness
2. Apologies and promises
3. Hope
4. Sexual interaction

Adapted from: Walker (1984).

© 1999 Springer Publishing Company.

Weekly Behavior Inventory

Handout

Client name: _____ Date: _____

Please list the approximate number of times you have been involved in the events listed below during the last week. If you were the one slapped, etc., put the number of times. If you did the slapping, etc., put the number of times.

HAPPENED TO ME

Pinching ____
Slapping ____
Grabbing ____
Kicking ____
Punching ____
Hair pulling ____
Throwing things ____
Throwing mate or shoving ____
Hitting with physical object ____
Choking ____
Threat of or use of weapon ____
Burning ____
Sexual abuse ____
Destruction of property ____
Verbal abuse ____
Emotional abuse ____

I DID TO PARTNER

Pinching ____
Slapping ____
Grabbing ____
Kicking ____
Punching ____
Hair pulling ____
Throwing things ____
Throwing mate or shoving ____
Hitting with physical object ____
Choking ____
Threat of or use of weapon ____
Burning ____
Sexual abuse ____
Destruction of property ____
Verbal abuse ____
Emotional abuse ____
Acted assertively ____
Communicated effectively ____
Used time-out ____
Controlled angry behavior ____

I DID HOMEWORK ____

HAPPENED TO CHILDREN

Pinching ____
Slapping ____
Grabbing ____
Hair pulling ____
Kicking ____
Punching ____
Throwing child ____
Hitting with physical object ____
Scarring child ____
Use of weapon ____
Threat of use of weapon ____
Burning ____
Sexual abuse ____
Verbal abuse ____
Emotional abuse ____

I DID TO CHILDREN

Pinching ____
Slapping ____
Grabbing ____
Hair pulling ____
Kicking ____
Punching ____
Throwing child ____
Hitting with physical object ____
Scarring child ____
Use of weapon ____
Threat of use of weapon ____
Burning ____
Sexual abuse ____
Verbal abuse ____
Emotional abuse ____
Acted assertively ____
Communicated effectively ____
Used time-out ____
Controlled angry behavior ____
Spent quality time ____

**I DON'T FEEL SAFE
TALKING IN GROUP** ____

Alcohol and Abuse: What's the Connection?

Handout

Some people who hurt the ones they love have problems with alcohol. Some also have problems with other drugs, like pot, crack, and cocaine. Ours is a culture that often encourages the abuse of alcohol, as well as the display of aggression under its influence. For example, this type of situation is often portrayed in movies. Consequently, people under the influence sometimes do things impulsively they may not ordinarily do, while their judgment and control are further impaired.

People use chemicals for many different reasons. You need to list for yourself the reasons you use chemicals. Then, you need to identify whether alcohol causes you personally to become aggressive, or to impair your judgment. Major themes that are often revealed during this thought-and-listing process are:

1. **Social Drinking**—There may be friend and/or cultural pressure to use/abuse alcohol. Currently commercials even emphasize "Why Ask Why? . . . Have another beer."
2. **Habit**—Many people equate socializing with alcohol use. For others, they believe the only way to unwind is through drinking. Drinking then becomes routine.
3. **Psychological Dependency**—A psychological dependency occurs at a point when alcohol use is so established, it's hard to imagine doing without it. Perhaps by this stage, temporary attempts have been made to abstain.
4. **Physical Dependency**—In the later stages of dependency, withdrawal can have severe effects. Medical, legal, vocational, and family problems attributed to alcohol abuse likely have already indicated a problem with alcohol.

No one ever established a goal of developing an alcohol/drug problem. Alcohol use may precede abuse, and the abuse is often progressive. You need to ask yourself if you have ever conducted yourself under the influence in ways you have later regretted. If the answer is "yes," the next question must be how healthy it is to continue to use chemicals that impair your judgment? You need to think about whether you have ever experienced memory lapses or "black outs," or to consider if you have ever been told that you have an alcohol problem.

Any "yes" answers to these questions indicate that alcohol use has impaired your ability to be fully in control of your life. Remember the 100% rule regarding responsibility. Alcohol problems are progressive—without help, they get worse. Can you really be 100% committed to being in control, and continue to use alcohol or drugs?

Help is available through recovery programs. Referrals can be made to assist you in getting the help you need.

This handout was developed by Ken Marlow, LCSW, in San Diego, CA.

© 1999 Springer Publishing Company.

III

Communicating and Expressing Feelings

Weekly Behavior Inventory

Client name: _____   Date: _____

Please list the approximate number of times you have been involved in the events listed below during the last week. If you were the one slapped, etc., put the number of times. If you did the slapping, etc., put the number of times.

HAPPENED TO ME

Pinching _____
Slapping _____
Grabbing _____
Kicking _____
Punching _____
Hair pulling _____
Throwing things _____
Throwing mate or shoving _____
Hitting with physical object _____
Choking _____
Threat of or use of weapon _____
Burning _____
Sexual abuse _____
Destruction of property _____
Verbal abuse _____
Emotional abuse _____

HAPPENED TO CHILDREN

Pinching _____
Slapping _____
Grabbing _____
Hair pulling _____
Kicking _____
Punching _____
Throwing child _____
Hitting with physical object _____
Scarring child _____
Use of weapon _____
Threat of use of weapon _____
Burning _____
Sexual abuse _____
Verbal abuse _____
Emotional abuse _____

I DID TO PARTNER

Pinching _____
Slapping _____
Grabbing _____
Kicking _____
Punching _____
Hair pulling _____
Throwing things _____
Throwing mate or shoving _____
Hitting with physical object _____
Choking _____
Threat of or use of weapon _____
Burning _____
Sexual abuse _____
Destruction of property _____
Verbal abuse _____
Emotional abuse _____
Acted assertively _____
Communicated effectively _____
Used time-out _____
Controlled angry behavior _____

I DID TO CHILDREN

Pinching _____
Slapping _____
Grabbing _____
Hair pulling _____
Kicking _____
Punching _____
Throwing child _____
Hitting with physical object _____
Scarring child _____
Use of weapon _____
Threat of use of weapon _____
Burning _____
Sexual abuse _____
Verbal abuse _____
Emotional abuse _____
Acted assertively _____
Communicated effectively _____
Used time-out _____
Controlled angry behavior _____
Spent quality time _____

I DID HOMEWORK _____

I DON'T FEEL SAFE TALKING IN GROUP _____

"Fair-Fighting" Rules

Handout

1. **Ask for an appointment for the discussion.**
   a. Set a mutually agreed on time.
   b. Set a mutually agreed on place.
   c. Determine the approximate duration.
   d. Advise regarding content.

2. **Do not argue "below the belt."**
   a. Don't call each other names, direct or indirect.
   b. Don't call each other's friends or family names, direct or indirect.
   c. Don't threaten, verbally or nonverbally.
   d. Don't use physical violence.

3. **Use "I" messages.**
   a. Example of "you" messages.
      • Promotes defensiveness.
      • Gives away power.
      • Gives responsibility to the other person.
   b. Example of "I" messages
      • Reduces defensiveness.
      • Retains control.
      • Shows acceptance of responsibility.

4. **Deal with feelings first.**
   a. Express your feelings
      • Become aware of what you are feeling.
      • Label what you are feeling.
      • Verbalize and describe what you feel.
   b. Listen
      • Be aware of what the other person is feeling through verbal and nonverbal cues.
      • Label the feelings so you can proceed accordingly.
      • Accept his or her right to feel what he or she wants to feel.

5. **Check that you are correctly labeling the other's feelings.**
   a. Words
   b. Nonverbal cues
   c. Check for incongruities.
   d. Be aware of thoughts and mind-reading.

6. **Ask for specific action.**
   a. Ask for what you want in detail.
   b. Ask what he or she wants; get details.
   c. Compromise and negotiate.

"Fair-Fighting" Rules *(Continued)*

Handout

7. **Take a time-out, if needed.**
   a. Know when to take a time-out.
   b. Know how to take a time-out.
   c. Mutually agree on when and how to take a time-out.
   d. Agree on the next appointment.

8. **Use teamwork.**
   a. Don't use fair fighting as a weapon or as a competition.
   b. Work together to use the rules.

9. **Never give up.**

Adapted from Bach & Wyden (1970).

"Dirty Fighter's" Instruction Manual*

INTRODUCTION

Not only can dirty fighting be a casual interest, a pleasant pastime, and a creative outlet, but many find it a way of life. Besides adding hours of excitement and entertainment to an otherwise drab existence, with dirty fighting one can obtain what people want most but are often least able to get: Their own way.

Although fighting dirty is practiced as a matter of course in homes and offices, at school, and at play, it is often thought that our ability to engage in underhanded warfare is natural and that no particular attention need be paid to developing one's abilities in this endeavor. All people do not come to the arena of human interaction equally equipped to do battle, however. On the contrary, many people find themselves unnecessarily crippled by moral, ethical, and temperamental biases that inhibit self-expression and leave them to face the world with a profound disadvantage. To make matters worse, our educational system has largely ignored this important area. It is for this reason, in an effort to make up for this unfortunate deficit, that this modest work has been created.

SOME GENERAL CONSIDERATIONS

Setting the Proper Tone

Like choosing the right timing, setting the proper tone is crucially important to getting a good argument going. Develop the ability to be hostile, ornery, unpredictable, or to throw temper tantrums and sulk for days when necessary. It is important also to learn the proper use of sarcasm, disapproving looks, exasperated sighs, and so on. Once an argument has started, move to the approach that will be most effective. Shouting and screaming are favorites for many, with occasional threats and intimidating remarks thrown in for emphasis. Although some people find that becoming hysterical usually produces the desired result, others prefer to let the partner be the one to get hysterical. In any case, be sure to follow through with statements such as, "If I had known you'd get so upset, I wouldn't have brought it up in the first place," or "Obviously you can't control yourself, so there's no point in discussing it any further."

Develop the Proper Attitude

There are a number of circumstances that automatically qualify you as being right and/or justified. The following are a few lead-ins that can be used to get you started on the right track:

1. **Family Wage-Earner**—"I'm working to pay for it, so the discussion is over."
2. **Person in Authority**—"That's the way things are. If you don't like it, that's just too bad. As long as you're here, you'll do what I tell you to do."
3. **Friend**—"I wouldn't think of bothering you unless I really needed your help. I'll really be hurt if you refuse."

---

* *Note:* **These are negative techniques that are often used in relationships—they are presented in this manner to exaggerate and point out their inappropriateness.**

"Dirty Fighter's" Instruction Manual *(Continued)*

4. **Loved One**—"I shouldn't have to ask you to do things for me. You should know how I feel without my having to tell you."
5. **Parent** (with children)—"I'm your father (or mother) and I know what's best for you."

The Importance of Good Timing

Many potentially lethal dirty fighters miss golden opportunities because they are unaware of the value of proper timing. Begin an argument just before your husband leaves for work. Argue with your wife at bedtime after a tiring day or when she has to get up early the next morning. Pester your children with household chores or homework just as they sit down to watch their favorite TV program or before they go out to play. In general, keep in mind that it is best to attack others when their guard is down, when they least expect it, or when they are least able to defend themselves.

Developing a Winning Style

Many people win arguments not because they are right, but because they have a style of arguing that is unbeatable. Choose the style that best suits your personality.

1. **Monopolize the conversation**—Don't let anyone get a word in edgewise. If the other person tries to speak, either ignore him or her completely or accuse him or her of cutting you off before you are finished.
2. **Meander**—Make short stories long, make mountains out of molehills, talk about things that are irrelevant to the issue. Do not, under any circumstances, come to the point.
3. **Don't listen**—While the other person is talking, use the time productively to think about how you are going to answer back. When it is your turn, ignore any and all concerns that may have been mentioned and go right to the points you would like to make.
4. **Be a problem solver**—This style is useful when the main concern is the other person's feelings. The approach here is to ignore the feelings and simply hand down decisions, solutions, or suggestions. Once you have offered a solution, that's all that needs to said, and the issue is closed.

SOME SPECIFIC TECHNIQUES

Collect Injustices

Collect slights, hurts, injustices, inequities, and let your anger build up to the point where you explode over relatively minor issues. Then, when you've had enough, shout, scream, terrorize, even threaten. You will be surprised to learn how good it feels getting things off your chest. An added benefit of collecting injustices is that you then rationalize almost anything you later wish to do, like getting a divorce, quitting your job, or having an affair.

"Dirty Fighter's" Instruction Manual (*Continued*)

Help with a Vengeance

There are countless opportunities to give advice, tell people what they should do, how they should feel, what they should think, all in the interest of being helpful. It doesn't matter whether or not they have asked your opinion; go ahead and give others the benefit of your experience. If someone should object to your unsolicited suggestions, point out to this person that you are only saying these things for his or her own good and that he or she should be able to accept constructive criticism.

Don't Get Mad, Get Even

Anger expressed openly can be uncomfortable for all concerned, so learn to find other ways to channel your feelings. Get revenge by sulking, having an affair, going on shopping sprees, rejecting the other sexually, and so on. In general, it is always a good idea to find ways to undermine the other's confidence or independence, because this tends to increase the effectiveness of your anger.

When the Going Gets Tough, the Tough Get Going

If the other person is saying something you don't like, it is time to get going. Walk out of the room, clam up, refuse to talk about it; when arguing with children, send them to their rooms. No need to hang around an unpleasant situation. No matter how much the other person feels his or her complaint is justified, no issue is so important that it can't be walked away from. Better yet, refuse to acknowledge that the situation even exists.

Play Psychiatrist

This is closely related to the previous technique, but it extends the concept somewhat. Analyze others, point out their shortcomings, their "hang-ups" and, where possible, explain in psychological terms the weaknesses you see in their character. Example: "You have a mother complex," or "The reason you say that is because you are basically insecure." The real secret in playing psychiatrist, however, involves the skillful use of labels. For instance: "You're an egomaniac," or a "dominating bitch." With a little forethought you can find a label for any behavior you don't like. If someone is drinking to relax, he or she is a "potential alcoholic;" if the person doesn't want sex, he or she is "frigid" or "impotent." By the way, if the person objects to your clinical evaluation, it is undoubtedly because he or she has an "inferiority complex" or "can't face the truth."

Devastate with Humor

Keep in mind that the most devastating remarks are often said in jest. Therefore, tease and humor your opponent. Be sarcastic but always smile to show that it's all in good fun. If the other person begins to get defensive, you can accuse him or her of being overly sensitive. This is an excellent tactic to use in public, because it shows that you are a fun-loving person with a sense of humor and that the other person is a spoilsport.

"Dirty Fighter's" Instruction
Manual *(Continued)*

Play One Person Against the Other

When out with your partner, always take long wistful looks at passing strangers of the opposite sex. Compare the success of others to those of your partner. A parent should never miss a chance to hold up the accomplishments of one child to another. A child should likewise never miss an opportunity to play one parent against the other.

Play the Martyr

Go out of your way to sacrifice your pleasure for others, even to the point of letting others take advantage of you. Later, when you want to get your way, preface your remarks with statements like: "How could you do this to me after all of the things I've done for you?" or "See how I've suffered because of you." You will be amazed at the power a little guilt gives you. The possibilities here are limitless.

Never Back Down

Backing down can only be considered a sign of weakness by the opposition. Right or wrong, you have to stand up for yourself. If you don't who else will? By the way, when was the last time you were wrong about something anyway?

Never Accept an Apology

Just because someone has said he or she is sorry, right away you are expected to forget about the wrong done to you. Never let the other person think he or she is forgiven. How else will he or she remember the next time? Learn to hold grudges, for years if necessary. A person's misconduct can be thrown up to him or her over and over again, giving you a decided edge in future disagreements.

Put the Other Person in a Double Bind

Criticize your spouse for gaining a little weight, not keeping up his or her appearance, and the like. Then, when he or she dresses up and looks especially good, accuse him or her of trying to impress people or flirting. Hound your children about hanging around the house too much. Then, when they are getting ready to go out to play, remind them of some chore they were supposed to do or tell them it's too close to supper. The idea is damned if you do, damned if you don't. Double binds artfully used can and do literally drive people crazy.

Chinese Water-Torture Technique

This heading is a grab-bag for a number of techniques that are meant to exasperate the opposition. Here are a few possibilities; make up your own variations:

1. **Be a chronic forgetter**—Never keep a promise; forget to do an errand. Act surprised when the other person gets upset as if to imply it didn't matter anyway. Forgetting birthdays and anniversaries also adds a nice touch, as does forgetting to call when you are delayed.

"Dirty Fighter's" Instruction Manual *(Continued)*

2. **Be a procrastinator**—Delay carrying out promises or obligations. The more others are depending on you, of course, the better. If there is a complaint, take the tack: "What are you getting excited about? I said I would do it, didn't I?" or "You're always nagging me about something; no wonder I never have a chance to get anything done." Being a procrastinator makes you look good because it gives the impression that you have so many important things to do that you don't have a chance to get all the trivial things done as well.

Note: "Important" means important to you; "trivial" means important to the other person.

The Kitchen-Sink Technique

Throw everything into the argument but the kitchen sink. No need to stick to the issue at hand; now is the time to bring up all the other incidents that have been bothering you. Talk about his or her past failings or defects in character, past injustices, unsettled issues from the last argument, and so on. Before long, so many irrelevant issues will have been brought up that the other person will begin to feel that winning an argument with you is next to impossible.

Ambush—The Art of Getting the Other Person Into a Corner

Be on the lookout for situations you can capitalize on later. Go through your spouse's wallet, listen in on the telephone extension, quiz your children's friends to find out what your kids have been up to. You will be amazed to find how much ammunition you can gather for your next fight. Once you have become proficient in this tactic, others will think twice about bringing up even the most legitimate grievance.

Note: Excerpts from *The "Dirty Fighter's" Instruction Manual* are reprinted with permission by Alan L. Summers, Transactional Dynamics Institute, Glenside, PA.

Weekly Behavior Inventory

Handout

Client name: _____ Date: _____

Please list the approximate number of times you have been involved in the events listed below during the last week. If you were the one slapped, etc., put the number of times. If you did the slapping, etc., put the number of times.

HAPPENED TO ME

Pinching ____
Slapping ____
Grabbing ____
Kicking ____
Punching ____
Hair pulling ____
Throwing things ____
Throwing mate or shoving ____
Hitting with physical object ____
Choking ____
Threat of or use of weapon ____
Burning ____
Sexual abuse ____
Destruction of property ____
Verbal abuse ____
Emotional abuse ____

I DID TO PARTNER

Pinching ____
Slapping ____
Grabbing ____
Kicking ____
Punching ____
Hair pulling ____
Throwing things ____
Throwing mate or shoving ____
Hitting with physical object ____
Choking ____
Threat of or use of weapon ____
Burning ____
Sexual abuse ____
Destruction of property ____
Verbal abuse ____
Emotional abuse ____
Acted assertively ____
Communicated effectively ____
Used time-out ____
Controlled angry behavior ____

I DID HOMEWORK ____

HAPPENED TO CHILDREN

Pinching ____
Slapping ____
Grabbing ____
Hair pulling ____
Kicking ____
Punching ____
Throwing child ____
Hitting with physical object ____
Scarring child ____
Use of weapon ____
Threat of use of weapon ____
Burning ____
Sexual abuse ____
Verbal abuse ____
Emotional abuse ____

I DID TO CHILDREN

Pinching ____
Slapping ____
Grabbing ____
Hair pulling ____
Kicking ____
Punching ____
Throwing child ____
Hitting with physical object ____
Scarring child ____
Use of weapon ____
Threat of use of weapon ____
Burning ____
Sexual abuse ____
Verbal abuse ____
Emotional abuse ____
Acted assertively ____
Communicated effectively ____
Used time-out ____
Controlled angry behavior ____
Spent quality time ____

I DON'T FEEL SAFE
TALKING IN GROUP ____

Family Communication Rules

Counselors may explain all the following rules to clients, or use only those that are appropriate for a particular couple.

> **Rule 1:** Actions speak louder than words, or nonverbal communication is more powerful than verbal communication.

People always send two messages when they communicate. They send a verbal message and a nonverbal message. The verbal is what you say with words. The nonverbal is what your body, voice, and physical mannerisms indicate. This includes facial expressions, gestures, tone of voice, and so on. Because there are so many nonverbal ways to communicate, it is very difficult, if impossible, not to communicate.

Example   A contradictory, inconsistent, or double message—A husband comes in the door after work and his wife is sitting on the sofa with a sad look on her face and she does not speak. He says hello, gives her a kiss, and asks if everything is okay. She responds by saying everything is fine, but she turns her face away and starts to cry.

When a family member sees or hears a contradictory or inconsistent message, the contradiction should be pointed out, discussed, and resolved.
(Think of examples and role play both inconsistent and contradictory messages.)

Example   If a wife feels that her husband is giving one message verbally but another with his body posture or facial expression, she should question this. A way of doing this might be to say, "Honey, you're saying that you feel okay, but your face looks flushed. You look really tense and you seem very quiet. Is there anything you want to talk about?"

Sometimes it is helpful to practice communication before a mirror, paying particular attention to nonverbal messages and contradictions.

> **Rule 2:** Define what is important and emphasize it; define what is unimportant and ignore it.

One of the main problems with this rule is that few couples can find a topic that can be labeled unimportant. This rule covers faultfinding. When criticism is always used, it is called faultfinding and leads to destructive consequences in a family relationship. What is important would be constructive criticism from some concerned and loving partners who can express this in a nondestructive manner. Criticism is a necessary and important part of helping another person grow as a human being. Destructive criticism is just what the term implies, and one needs to decide the type of criticism he or she is going to give *before* giving it. Timing is an important factor because any criticism, at certain periods of stress, will not be accepted.

Couples who have trouble determining the differences between important and unimportant issues can have counselors examine the issues one by one to help agree on the classification. They must then stick to the agreed-on important topics and not refer to the unimportant matters. Problem-solving techniques will work in this area.

Family Communication Rules *(Continued)*

Handout

Example   "I'm so angry because you never talk to me, you don't help around the house, you always squeeze the toothpaste from the bottom of the tube, and you never smile at my mother."

It is important to decide what the major problem areas are and separate them from the picky areas of faultfinding.

Rule 3:	Be clear and specific in communication.

Being clear and specific in communication is especially important in problem solving. Some people tend to be very vague in their statements. A problem that is stated vaguely is less likely to be solved than a problem that is stated clearly. The following are suggestions to help ensure clear, specific communications:

1. **Discuss one problem at a time.**

   Some people tend to bring up a number of problems at one time. The more problems that are talked about at one time, the less likely it is that any of them will be solved.

Example   If the main issue that you want to solve is getting the rest of the family to help with household chores, then don't bring up other issues. "You and the children never help around the house. I know you don't like my mother, and you are never affectionate to me anymore."

2. **Avoid vagueness or generalities.**

   Define and clarify the terms and expression you use, and ask your partner to define and clarify his or her terms and expressions.

Example   "I don't like your **attitude**." (Clarify attitude.)
            "You're never **nice** to my mother." (Clarify nice.)
            "I want you to be more **romantic**." (Clarify what being more romantic would involve.)

3. **Do not accept the use of vague words by your partner.**

   Again, ask for feedback and clarity from your partner. Even one vague word in a confrontation with someone can lead to an argument, as meanings become lost through personal perception and interpretation. This perception of the other person's intent may or may not be accurate so probing is needed.

Example   "I'm feeling real **bummed out**." (Check this out by asking the person what they mean by "bummed out.")
            "You **hurt** me." (How did I hurt you? What did I do that hurt you?)
            "You're acting **hostile**." (What am I doing that makes you think I'm acting hostile?)

Family Communication Rules *(Continued)*

> **Rule 4:**   Test all your assumptions verbally. Get your partner's okay before you make a decision that involves them.

Testing your assumptions is critical in relationships. Some people consider the failure to test an assumption or failure to consult with them regarding a decision as rude and insulting.

Example   A wife is told by her husband that he has invited another couple for dinner. He has "assumed" his wife would not mind. In fact, she may become angry, because she was not consulted. A woman decides to rearrange the bedroom furniture. The husband feels that he has been ignored and that his opinion does not matter.

Here again, mind-reading comes into play. Find out what mind-reading is, if you do not already know. Play a game called "I know something you don't think I know." Each person guesses what the other is thinking by nonverbal clues only. List at least four feelings or thoughts you believe the other is feeling or thinking. These must be conveyed with nonverbal information. Then check the perception verbally. How accurate were you? Can you afford to be wrong even one time? It is important to ask questions.

> **Rule 5:**   Realize that each event can be seen from a different point of view.

One way to begin to discuss this rule is to check which sensory system each partner uses to relate to the environment and other people. These are visual (eye), auditory (ear), and kinesthetic (touch). Counselors can ask questions to help focus on which system is used most by the individuals. Then compare and see if they use the same system. If not, they can still communicate, but they must learn to use the other person's system to relate to him or her.

When a member of a family makes a statement from a perception that he or she believes to be true, another person may not agree because his or her interpretation of the situation presented is contrary to the first person's belief. When this happens, counselors need to draw attention to this discrepancy and have family members explain specifically what they mean.

> **Rule 6:**   Learn to disagree without destructive arguments.

A discussion is an exchange of ideas or feelings, in which the objective is to solve a problem or reach more understanding.

An argument is an expression of ideas and feelings, but the intentions are to hurt the partner or raise one's own self-esteem at the expense of the partner. Arguments are often accompanied by intense anger, nagging, or whining.

Some will avoid a disagreement for several reasons. These are fear of losing control, losing the argument, having faults exposed, not wanting to hurt the other, and so on.

Learning the Fair-Fighting Rules can help reduce some of these fears. For contrast, counselors can use the *Dirty Fighter's Manual* for a humorous opposing view. It must be emphasized that this is a tongue-in-cheek approach. Even if discussions do not lead to positive results, they are still better than an argument that leads to hurt feelings, unfair attacks, sarcasm, and humiliation, in which case no one gains.

Family Communication Rules *(Continued)*

Handout

Rule 7:   Be open and honest about your feelings.

It is not likely that family members will *always* be open and honest. When discussing this rule, the counselors need to offer explanations. First, not all subjects need to be discussed openly.

Example   "I don't like your hair, your face has too many pimples, your ears are too large, I have gas, and so on."

Second, some issues that are not discussed need to be brought into the open if they are indirectly leading to the problems.

Example   If one member is angry about something but only keeps it inside, he or she may take it out on others by overcriticizing a minor event. This can lead to inappropriate, angry outbursts. This can also result in other members "walking on eggs" for reasons they are not sure of.

Third, an honest expression of feelings will let others know exactly what is going on and even if no answers can be found, at least the others are aware of the problem. A definition of the problem is the first step toward solving it, and this can be pointed out to the clients.

Rule 8:   Let the effect, not the intention, of your communication be your guide.

Often an unintentional hurtful comment can be made, and when the person realizes this, a countercomment such as "I didn't mean it" or "I was only kidding" does not solve the original hurt effect. This behavior will then influence the partner's perception of what is being communicated in future discussions. It is important for the one who is hurting the other to realize what the effect has been and that he or she created the hurt feelings. The intention of a comment must be in harmony with the actual verbal communication. When this problem is witnessed by the counselors, they need to bring attention to it and try to help create a clarification of effect and intent.

Rule 9:   Do not preach or lecture.

With children, lecturing can have its usefulness, but with teenagers and adults the benefits are limited. Little needs to be said about this rule except that lectures and sermons are generally destructive. They result in defensiveness or low self-esteem. If problems arise, the best course for counselors is to teach problem-solving techniques found in the session about problem solving.

Rule 10: Do not use excuses or fall for excuses.

The difference between excuses and reasons is the important aspect of this rule. A legitimate reason for being late is better than a made-up excuse. Excuses are used for repeated inconsiderate acts whether a family member, a boss, a coworker, or a friend is involved. Such statements (i.e.,

Family Communication Rules *(Continued)*

running out of gas) can be a reason if it happened once. It is an excuse if it happens over and over. Accepting excuses can lead to resentment and unresolved feelings of conflict and hostility.

Parents use excuses when communicating with their children, thereby teaching them to use excuses themselves. Parents will make excuses to the child when they are reluctant to give the real reason for saying "no" to a certain request.

Excuses are often rationalized and designed to fool the user him/herself. At the other end of the spectrum are excuses to protect him/herself from some unpleasant consequence. Many times both partners are aware of the invalidity of the excuse, but they say nothing. This allows some resentment or anger to develop that will one day surface in an argument or it may even be the reason for the argument.

> **Rule 11:** Learn when to use humor and when to be serious. Do not subject your partner to destructive teasing.

Humor when appropriately used is an important emotional resource. Humor clears the air and bring relief from pent-up tensions. Humor is pleasant, and people enjoy laughing with the one who elicits the humor. Humor can be destructive, however. This can occur when it is directed toward another for the purpose of making fun of the other person. Using humor to avoid an uncomfortable situation, when in reality the situation needs to be dealt with, is another time when humor is inappropriate.

There is an expression called "kid serious," which means that someone makes a hurting comment directed at another person and then follows that comment with "I was only kidding." The humor is lost and the hurt is all that is left. Kid serious is a game many play and it leads to hurt, anger, and resentment. Counselors need to point this out whenever it is observed and give other examples to clients. Role play can be used here. Kid serious robs communication of clarity and honesty, and it results in lowered self-esteem.

Teasing is another form of humor that can be destructive, depending on the intent and the person to whom it is directed. Children can tease each other and have fun; but when one teases another into doing something that will get the child in trouble, then the teasing becomes a problem. In general, teasing another about things over which he or she has no control (such as the shape of a nose, length of legs, etc.) and teasing for the purpose of making another do something he or she does not want to do should be avoided.

Weekly Behavior Inventory

Handout

Client name: _____   Date: _____

Please list the approximate number of times you have been involved in the events listed below during the last week. If you were the one slapped, etc., put the number of times. If you did the slapping, etc., put the number of times.

HAPPENED TO ME

Pinching _____
Slapping _____
Grabbing _____
Kicking _____
Punching _____
Hair pulling _____
Throwing things _____
Throwing mate or shoving _____
Hitting with physical object _____
Choking _____
Threat of or use of weapon _____
Burning _____
Sexual abuse _____
Destruction of property _____
Verbal abuse _____
Emotional abuse _____

I DID TO PARTNER

Pinching _____
Slapping _____
Grabbing _____
Kicking _____
Punching _____
Hair pulling _____
Throwing things _____
Throwing mate or shoving _____
Hitting with physical object _____
Choking _____
Threat of or use of weapon _____
Burning _____
Sexual abuse _____
Destruction of property _____
Verbal abuse _____
Emotional abuse _____
Acted assertively _____
Communicated effectively _____
Used time-out _____
Controlled angry behavior _____

I DID HOMEWORK _____

HAPPENED TO CHILDREN

Pinching _____
Slapping _____
Grabbing _____
Hair pulling _____
Kicking _____
Punching _____
Throwing child _____
Hitting with physical object _____
Scarring child _____
Use of weapon _____
Threat of use of weapon _____
Burning _____
Sexual abuse _____
Verbal abuse _____
Emotional abuse _____

I DID TO CHILDREN

Pinching _____
Slapping _____
Grabbing _____
Hair pulling _____
Kicking _____
Punching _____
Throwing child _____
Hitting with physical object _____
Scarring child _____
Use of weapon _____
Threat of use of weapon _____
Burning _____
Sexual abuse _____
Verbal abuse _____
Emotional abuse _____
Acted assertively _____
Communicated effectively _____
Used time-out _____
Controlled angry behavior _____
Spent quality time _____

I DON'T FEEL SAFE TALKING IN GROUP _____

"I" Messages

"I" messages are specific, nonjudgmental, and focus on the speaker. In contrast, "you" messages are hostile, blaming, and focus on the other person and cause him or her to feel attacked. Reframing "you" messages into "I" messages can help you communicate because the other person will not feel attacked. Being attacked and blamed makes most of us put up our defenses and get ready to fight.

To construct an "I" message:

1. Describe the **behavior** that is affecting you.
   (Just describe, don't blame.)
2. State your **feelings** about the consequence the behavior produces in you.
3. State the **consequence.**

An easy formula to construct "I" messages uses these phrases:

1. When you (state the behavior), _____,
2. I feel (state the feeling),_____,
3. Because (state the consequences), _____.

Note: Stressing the word "because" can help by more strongly connecting the feeling and consequence elements of the message. This minimizes blame and keeps the focus on you.

The parts of an "I" message do not have to be delivered in order, and sometimes the inclusion of the feeling statement is not necessary. The important thing to remember is to keep the focus on you and avoid placing blame.

EXAMPLES

1. When you take long phone calls during dinner, I get angry because I begin to think you don't want to talk to me.
2. When you don't come home or call, I get scared because I'm afraid something has happened to you.
3. When you yell at me when things are hectic, I get so rattled that I end up making more mistakes.

Effective Expression and Listening

Handout

EFFECTIVE EXPRESSION

1. **Messages should be direct.**
   A. Know when something needs to be said. Don't assume that people know what you want or think.
   B. Don't be afraid to say how you feel or to ask for what you want. Avoid hinting.

   Example   During commercials a husband keeps asking if the movie is almost over, hoping his wife will get the hint that he wants her to spend time with him.

2. **Messages should be immediate.**
   A. Anger has a way of smoldering and building up; it may then come out in aggressive ways.
   B. There are two main advantages of immediate communications:

   * People are more apt to learn what you want and to make efforts to meet those needs or wants.
   * Intimacy increases because you are sharing your responses.

3. **Messages should be clear.**
   A. Don't ask questions when you need to make a statement.

   Example   "Do we really need to go to that party?" What may be meant is that the person doesn't really want to go.

   B. Make sure what you say verbally matches the nonverbal messages you might be giving. Avoid double messages.

   Example   You tell your spouse he needs to get out of the house more instead of sitting around watching TV. When he does get out of the house, however, you accuse him of always running off and leaving you to do everything at home.

Role Play

Practice saying "Right now I feel _____." and "Right now I want _____." Do this several times. Also, give feedback about what your partner has said and what you saw in your partner's nonverbal cues, such as tone of voice, eye contact, or how he or she holds his or her body while speaking.

   C. Distinguish between observations and thoughts. Determine what is happening (the facts) as opposed to your judgments, theories, beliefs, or opinions.
   D. Focus on one thing at a time. Stick with a topic. Don't jump around. It may be confusing as to why you are upset or what you want.

4. **Messages should be supportive.**
   A. Supportive messages are a way of honestly saying how you feel and what you want without intentionally devastating the other person.
   B. Ways of hurting someone:

   * Using labels such as you're stupid, lazy, evil, cruel, and so on
   * Using sarcasm
   * Dragging up the past
   * Using negative comparisons

Effective Expression and Listening *(Continued)*

- Using judgmental "you" messages: you never help me anymore
- Using threats: you threaten to leave or get a divorce

ACTIVE LISTENING

1. **Mirroring**
   A. Active listening or mirroring involves paraphrasing. Paraphrasing is stating in your own words what you think the other person has said.
   B. Active listening is a communication technique that enables you to be certain you understand what the other person is saying. It can also be used to make sure the other person understands what you are trying to say.
   C. Some lead-ins used in mirroring are:

   - What I hear you saying is . . .
   - In other words . . .
   - What happened was . . .
   - Do you mean . . .

2. **Clarifying**
   A. Clarifying is basically asking questions to get more information.
   B. Clarifying also lets the other person know you are interested in what he or she is saying.

3. **Feedback**
   A. Feedback is letting your spouse know about your perceptions, reactions, and what is happening inside you concerning the situation or discussion at hand.
   B. Feedback helps the other person know the effect of his or her communication. This allows the opportunity to clarify any error or misunderstanding in the communication.
   C. Feedback should be immediate, honest, and supportive.

Role Play

Talk to your partner and use the types of phrases that follow. Give time for your partner to respond.

"I notice (body gesture or expression) and I wonder what that means."

Example   "I noticed that you slammed the door and kicked the cat when you came in and I wonder what that means."

"I notice (body gesture or expression) and I am afraid it means _____."

Example   "I notice that your body posture is stiff, your legs and arms are crossed and you refuse to make eye contact with me, and I am afraid it means that you are angry with me."

Clear up any ambiguity and talk about what you meant to communicate.

Effective Expression and Listening *(Continued)*

4. **Empathy**
   A. Empathy means trying to understand what the person is feeling. This does not mean that you agree.
   B. Try to understand what danger the person might be experiencing, what he or she is asking for, and what need is producing the emotion (i.e., anger).

5. **Openness**
   A. Listen without judging or finding fault.
   B. Try to see the other person's point of view. This does not mean you have to agree.
   C. Listen to the whole statement; don't make premature evaluations.

6. **Awareness**
   A. How does the information being communicated fit with known facts?
   B. Listen and look for agreement between what is being said and the nonverbal expressions that are present.

Note: **Some keys to being a good listener:** Have good eye contact, lean slightly forward, reinforce by nodding or paraphrasing, clarify by asking questions, avoid distractions, try to understand empathetically what was said.

Six Blocks to Listening

1. **Comparing**—How someone measures up.
   Example   Direct—"You've been on your job just as long as Bill has, but he's a supervisor."
   Less Direct—"Don't those tall men look so lean and handsome." (Your partner is short and broad.)

2. **Mind-Reading**—Assume you know what the person is thinking or feeling.
   Example   "I know what you're thinking. You're afraid if I go do anything that I'm going to flirt with women."

3. **Filtering**—Selective listening. Does not hear all that is said.
   Example   After an evening out, the wife says to the husband, "Really fun evening, the restaurant was nice, but the drive was too long." All the husband heard was the last comment about the drive, he took it as a negative put-down, and says, "You never want to have a good time with me; you are never happy."

4. **Identifying**—This means referring everything to your own experience.
   Example   Someone is trying to tell you about a problem with his or her boss and you start telling him or her about your problems.

5. **Advising**—Problem solving without permission.
   Example   A woman comes in and tells husband about a problem at work. He immediately gives her a laid out plan of action. All she wanted was for him to listen.

6. **Being Right**—Wanting to win.
   Example   Seeing every discussion as an opportunity to win instead of trying to compromise; making excuses if you can't win.

Talk about which of these blocks to listening you use. You can role play some of these in Group.

Weekly Behavior Inventory

Handout

Client name: _____ Date: _____

Please list the approximate number of times you have been involved in the events listed below during the last week. If you were the one slapped, etc., put the number of times. If you did the slapping, etc., put the number of times.

HAPPENED TO ME

Pinching _____
Slapping _____
Grabbing _____
Kicking _____
Punching _____
Hair pulling _____
Throwing things _____
Throwing mate or shoving _____
Hitting with physical object _____
Choking _____
Threat of or use of weapon _____
Burning _____
Sexual abuse _____
Destruction of property _____
Verbal abuse _____
Emotional abuse _____

HAPPENED TO CHILDREN

Pinching _____
Slapping _____
Grabbing _____
Hair pulling _____
Kicking _____
Punching _____
Throwing child _____
Hitting with physical object _____
Scarring child _____
Use of weapon _____
Threat of use of weapon _____
Burning _____
Sexual abuse _____
Verbal abuse _____
Emotional abuse _____

I DID TO PARTNER

Pinching _____
Slapping _____
Grabbing _____
Kicking _____
Punching _____
Hair pulling _____
Throwing things _____
Throwing mate or shoving _____
Hitting with physical object _____
Choking _____
Threat of or use of weapon _____
Burning _____
Sexual abuse _____
Destruction of property _____
Verbal abuse _____
Emotional abuse _____
Acted assertively _____
Communicated effectively _____
Used time-out _____
Controlled angry behavior _____

I DID HOMEWORK _____

I DID TO CHILDREN

Pinching _____
Slapping _____
Grabbing _____
Hair pulling _____
Kicking _____
Punching _____
Throwing child _____
Hitting with physical object _____
Scarring child _____
Use of weapon _____
Threat of use of weapon _____
Burning _____
Sexual abuse _____
Verbal abuse _____
Emotional abuse _____
Acted assertively _____
Communicated effectively _____
Used time-out _____
Controlled angry behavior _____
Spent quality time _____

**I DON'T FEEL SAFE
TALKING IN GROUP** _____

Handling Criticism

Everyone is occasionally criticized by someone. No one is perfect. How you handle criticism is especially important in intimate relationships. It is not uncommon to react (respond) defensively to critical observations.

Typical responses to criticism are:

NEGATIVE

1. **Avoid the criticism or critic.** Ignore, change the subject, make jokes (be funny), refuse to talk about it, be too busy, withdraw, or even walk away.

    Examples   When someone says something critical to you, don't respond verbally, just give the person a "go to hell" look, and walk out of the room.

    When the other person is talking to you, look at the floor, stare into space, or just look through the person. Avoid making direct eye contact.

    Make statements indicating that you are just "too busy" to deal with the person right now. "Okay, get with me later, I'm late for an important meeting."

    "I don't want to talk about this: Subject closed!"

    Your boss is upset because you were drunk at the party last night and really acted crazy. Make light of what he is saying by saying, "Yeah, did you see me dancing on that table with a bucket on my head?"

    Suppose you are late for work and your boss confronts you. You could change the subject by talking about how you're going to have to get your car fixed so it will be more reliable.

2. **Deny the critical comment.** Deny facts, argue, present evidence, do not entertain the idea of accepting anything.

    Examples   Argue about what the facts are. Fight about all the minor details.

    "No, I wasn't late on Monday, I think it was Tuesday."

    "No, I didn't call your mother a toad, I said she was always croaking about something."

    Deny that it happened: "I wasn't drunk at the party."

3. **Make excuses.** Explain your behavior in detail, be very sorry, have an alibi or excuse, or argue the importance of your behavior.

    Examples   You were late to pick your spouse up, so you go into detail about how the keys got lost, you had to search for them, and the baby is always losing everything. Your spouse will soon just want to forget he or she ever said anything.

    Again, you are late and your spouse is upset: "Well, it was just a movie, look at all the important things I have to take care of everyday."

    "So I had my tongue in her ear at the party, that doesn't mean I care about her. You know you're the only one for me."

Handling Criticism *(Continued)*

Handout

4. **Fight Back.** Attack, get even, the best defense is the best offense, fight fire with fire.

   Examples   Suppose a family member says something about you gaining weight. Attack this person's weight, housekeeping, handwriting, parenting skills, and so on. or you can get even by burning the meal or being late when he or she really wanted to be somewhere on time.

POSITIVE

1. **Ask for details.** Criticisms are often vague or given in generalities. "You're lazy" or "I don't like the way you're acting." When you ask for details you find out exactly what the other person is talking about. When you ask for details try to find out who, what, where, when, and how.

   Examples   **Who** do I pick on?

   Exactly **what** did I do that hurt your feelings?

   When was I late?

   Where did this take place?

   Why do you think I don't consider your feelings?

   How do I act when you say I bore you?

2. **Agree with the accurate part of the criticism.** A second step to handling criticism effectively is to agree with the part of the criticism that is true. Even if you feel the other person is completely wrong, you can use two types of agreement statements.

   A. Agree with the truth. Agree with the accurate part of what is being said.

   - Do not put yourself down.
   - You do not have to agree to change.
   - Do not defend yourself.
   - Use self-disclosure instead of self-defense.
   - Watch for generalities in the criticism.
   - Listen, attend, and monitor.

   Example   Your spouse says, "You were rude to my mother." Respond, "Yes, I was rude to her that one time when I said her red dress looked like a gunny sack."

   B. Agree with the critic's right to an opinion. This doesn't mean you have to agree with his or her opinion.

   - Avoid issues of right/wrong, good/bad, okay/not okay.
   - Use self-disclosure.
   - You do not have to defend your opinion, but you may wish to explain if possible.
   - Listen, attend, and monitor.

Handling Criticism *(Continued)*

Example   Suppose you go to a movie and you like the movie but the other person did not enjoy it. "I enjoyed the movie, I guess we have different tastes in movies." These agreement statements will decrease the chances of the person being defensive.

General guidelines for handling criticism

- Learn to see criticism as an opportunity to learn and grow.
- Try to avoid being defensive.
- Listen actively.
- Use attending behavior.
- Watch nonverbal language.
- Monitor physical and emotional cues.
- Act, do not react.

How to Offer Criticism

Handout

1. **Cool down.** Try to avoid offering criticism when you are too emotional. Wait until you have better control of your emotions.

2. **Consider your intent.** Realize the difference between constructive and destructive criticism. Is your intent to create a more positive relationship or zap your partner?

3. **Separate fact from fantasy.** Did your partner really use most of the gas in your car so that you would run out of gas in a bad part of town and be killed? Try to be rational.

4. **Do it now.** Try to offer criticism as soon after the act as possible. This will help you avoid saving up grievances for an emotional explosion in the future. Also, it is usually much easier to deal with something that just happened, rather than trusting a faulty memory.

5. **Make an appointment.** If you can't do it now, make an appointment to discuss it later. Both should agree on time, length of discussion, place, and content.

6. **Offer ideas, suggestions, and options.** It is helpful if you can offer possible solutions, constructive alternatives, or any ideas to solve the problem. Think of it as a team effort.

7. **Know when to be emotional, and when to be logical.** It is acceptable and healthy to talk about how you feel about a particular behavior; but when it comes to problem solving, it is generally best to be more logical.

8. **Do not play psychologist.** Try to limit comments regarding the causes, motives, or unconscious meaning of another person's behavior. Focus on the behavior and possible solutions to the problem.

9. **Be specific.** Avoid generalizations in criticism. No one can change unless he or she knows exactly what you want. Consider who, what, when, where, why, and how when you offer criticism.

10. **Praise in public, criticize in private.** No one likes to have his or her faults pointed out in front of an audience. On the other hand, most people won't object to a little public stroking.

11. **Praise more than you criticize.** It is okay to criticize, even necessary and productive if done correctly; but remember that people are more likely to respond favorably to criticism if they receive praise on a regular basis.

Weekly Behavior Inventory

Client name: _____   Date: _____

Please list the approximate number of times you have been involved in the events listed below during the last week. If you were the one slapped, etc., put the number of times. If you did the slapping, etc., put the number of times.

HAPPENED TO ME

Pinching ____
Slapping ____
Grabbing ____
Kicking ____
Punching ____
Hair pulling ____
Throwing things ____
Throwing mate or shoving ____
Hitting with physical object ____
Choking ____
Threat of or use of weapon ____
Burning ____
Sexual abuse ____
Destruction of property ____
Verbal abuse ____
Emotional abuse ____

HAPPENED TO CHILDREN

Pinching ____
Slapping ____
Grabbing ____
Hair pulling ____
Kicking ____
Punching ____
Throwing child ____
Hitting with physical object ____
Scarring child ____
Use of weapon ____
Threat of use of weapon ____
Burning ____
Sexual abuse ____
Verbal abuse ____
Emotional abuse ____

I DID TO PARTNER

Pinching ____
Slapping ____
Grabbing ____
Kicking ____
Punching ____
Hair pulling ____
Throwing things ____
Throwing mate or shoving ____
Hitting with physical object ____
Choking ____
Threat of or use of weapon ____
Burning ____
Sexual abuse ____
Destruction of property ____
Verbal abuse ____
Emotional abuse ____
Acted assertively ____
Communicated effectively ____
Used time-out ____
Controlled angry behavior ____

I DID TO CHILDREN

Pinching ____
Slapping ____
Grabbing ____
Hair pulling ____
Kicking ____
Punching ____
Throwing child ____
Hitting with physical object ____
Scarring child ____
Use of weapon ____
Threat of use of weapon ____
Burning ____
Sexual abuse ____
Verbal abuse ____
Emotional abuse ____
Acted assertively ____
Communicated effectively ____
Used time-out ____
Controlled angry behavior ____
Spent quality time ____

I DID HOMEWORK ____

I DON'T FEEL SAFE TALKING IN GROUP ____

How Do You Feel Today?

Handout

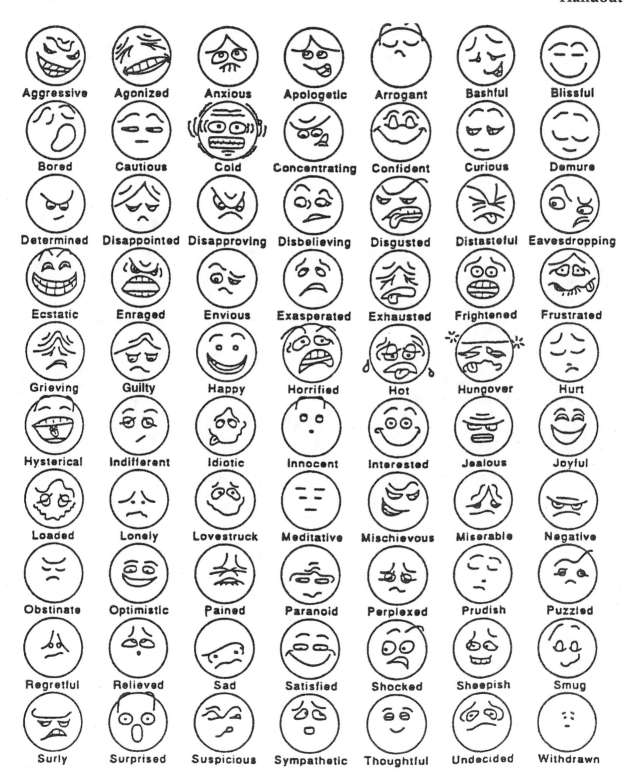

Aggressive Agonized Anxious Apologetic Arrogant Bashful Blissful

Bored Cautious Cold Concentrating Confident Curious Demure

Determined Disappointed Disapproving Disbelieving Disgusted Distasteful Eavesdropping

Ecstatic Enraged Envious Exasperated Exhausted Frightened Frustrated

Grieving Guilty Happy Horrified Hot Hungover Hurt

Hysterical Indifferent Idiotic Innocent Interested Jealous Joyful

Loaded Lonely Lovestruck Meditative Mischievous Miserable Negative

Obstinate Optimistic Pained Paranoid Perplexed Prudish Puzzled

Regretful Relieved Sad Satisfied Shocked Sheepish Smug

Surly Surprised Suspicious Sympathetic Thoughtful Undecided Withdrawn

Jealousy: Taming the Green-Eyed Monster

Handout

Jealousy is one of those emotions that can tie our stomach in knots in a hurry. A little bit of jealousy is natural, especially when we fear losing someone close to us. Jealousy becomes a problem when we spend too much energy worrying about losing a loved one, when we let jealousy build and we try to control another through aggression, or when we stifle a relationship by placing extreme restrictions on our partners.

Pete got himself really worked up whenever he went to a party with his wife, Sue. It seemed that she was attracted to some of the other men, and apparently they were attracted to her. Deep inside he was afraid that she would find another man more attractive and exciting than he was. He feared losing her love. But what usually happened after a party was a fight, a fight not about jealousy but about some other matter.

One day after one of these fights, Pete was thinking about how upset he made himself with jealousy. He tried to look at the situation in a more objective way—the way an outside observer would. After a while he was able to say to himself: "There are many aspects of my wife I find attractive. It is only natural that other men will sometimes find her attractive too. If that happens, it does not mean I will lose her. My fears and anger come from doubting my worth, not from other people's behavior and thoughts. If other men like my partner, then they agree with my opinion of her, and that's positive."

Joe's jealousy was even stronger than Pete's. He would question his wife at length when she came home, asking where she had been, who she had been with, and the details of her activities. He sometimes tore himself up wondering if she was having an affair. He would get urges to follow her everywhere or demand that she stay home. It seemed that the more he questioned her the more he disbelieved her.

It was after hearing his friend, Steve, talk about wanting to have an affair that he realized what was happening. The times when he was most suspicious of his wife were the times when he had sexual fantasies or romantic fantasies about other women. Now when he noticed jealousy, he asked himself, "Am I projecting my fantasies onto my partner because I'm feeling guilty about them?"

For many men, mentioning jealous feelings is not a cool thing to do—to admit jealousy is to admit a weakness. If, however, you view some jealousy as natural and as another "okay" emotion to share with your partner, both you and your partner can have the privilege of getting to know each other better.

Sally found the best way for her to "tame the monster" was to let her husband know she felt jealous. She felt very relieved being able to talk about the subject. Instead of responding with ridicule, her husband seemed to respect her more. Both of them went on to tell each other which of their partner's behaviors they could not tolerate—affairs, flirting, and so on. They were able to work out some contracts that specified the limits of the relationship.

What Pete, Joe, and Sally learned about taming jealousy was the following:

- Some jealousy is normal, and it's best to talk about it rather than hide it.
- I can choose to see my partner's attractiveness and behavior as either negative or positive—if I see it negatively, I am likely to upset myself and waste energy.
- It will help me to ask: "Is my jealousy coming from a projection of my own fantasies or behavior?"
- I have a right to request and contract for some **specific** limits on my partner's behavior (not thoughts), and my partner has the same right.

Adapted from *Alternatives to Aggression* by Daniel G. Saunders (1990).

Weekly Behavior Inventory

Handout

Client name: _____   Date: _____

Please list the approximate number of times you have been involved in the events listed below during the last week. If you were the one slapped, etc., put the number of times. If you did the slapping, etc., put the number of times.

HAPPENED TO ME

Pinching   _____
Slapping   _____
Grabbing   _____
Kicking   _____
Punching   _____
Hair pulling   _____
Throwing things   _____
Throwing mate or shoving   _____
Hitting with physical object   _____
Choking   _____
Threat of or use of weapon   _____
Burning   _____
Sexual abuse   _____
Destruction of property   _____
Verbal abuse   _____
Emotional abuse   _____

HAPPENED TO CHILDREN

Pinching   _____
Slapping   _____
Grabbing   _____
Hair pulling   _____
Kicking   _____
Punching   _____
Throwing child   _____
Hitting with physical object   _____
Scarring child   _____
Use of weapon   _____
Threat of use of weapon   _____
Burning   _____
Sexual abuse   _____
Verbal abuse   _____
Emotional abuse   _____

I DID TO PARTNER

Pinching   _____
Slapping   _____
Grabbing   _____
Kicking   _____
Punching   _____
Hair pulling   _____
Throwing things   _____
Throwing mate or shoving   _____
Hitting with physical object   _____
Choking   _____
Threat of or use of weapon   _____
Burning   _____
Sexual abuse   _____
Destruction of property   _____
Verbal abuse   _____
Emotional abuse   _____
Acted assertively   _____
Communicated effectively   _____
Used time-out   _____
Controlled angry behavior   _____

I DID HOMEWORK   _____

I DID TO CHILDREN

Pinching   _____
Slapping   _____
Grabbing   _____
Hair pulling   _____
Kicking   _____
Punching   _____
Throwing child   _____
Hitting with physical object   _____
Scarring child   _____
Use of weapon   _____
Threat of use of weapon   _____
Burning   _____
Sexual abuse   _____
Verbal abuse   _____
Emotional abuse   _____
Acted assertively   _____
Communicated effectively   _____
Used time-out   _____
Controlled angry behavior   _____
Spent quality time   _____

I DON'T FEEL SAFE TALKING IN GROUP   _____

Emotional Awareness and Expression

For each situation that follows:

- **Acknowledge your feelings.**
- **Identify the specific emotions felt.**
- **Describe the physical sensations are you having.**
- **Express how you feel by using "I feel" statements.**

Your spouse was going to meet you downtown for lunch, and you have been waiting over an hour. She finally arrives and says she had a few errands to run before she came.

You are visiting your mother-in-law and she says, "You've gained some weight, haven't you?" You are sensitive about your weight.

You are well qualified for a promotion, but your boss promotes his best friend who is not as qualified and has been there only a short time.

You are late getting home and your spouse demands an explanation, but as soon as you begin he/she interrupts and starts yelling and saying how inconsiderate you are.

Anger Styles

People have different ways of expressing anger. Understanding each other's anger style may make it easier for us to live with one another.

FIVE ANGER STYLES

1. **The Terrible-Tempered Mr. Bangs**   Anger is part of these people's daily lives. They have a tendency to take everything very personally and do not trust anyone. This type will run you off the road or swear at you if your driving displeases him.

2. **The Quiet Ones**   When these people get angry they tend to withdraw. They may not speak for days or might just mope around letting you guess what is going on. Even when asked, he or she may say very politely and coldly, "Nothing's wrong." This person's battle plan is to simulate "The Cold War."

3. **The Martyr**   These people may be very upset inside but not show any outward anger at all. They have a tendency to be indirect in their attack plan. They may be continually late or burn your favorite meal.

4. **The Hipshooter**   These people are quick to become angry, but get over it just as quickly. They may be impulsive, volatile, and wonder why the other person is still upset after they have already forgotten what they were upset about.

5. **The Counterattackers**   These people hide anger by being critical of others. They may give the message: "If you don't like me, I don't like you."

Decide what your anger styles are, and if any of the preceding types describes you. What about your partner?

Abusive-Incidents Graph
Physical—Verbal—Sexual

**Number of
Incidents
Per Week**

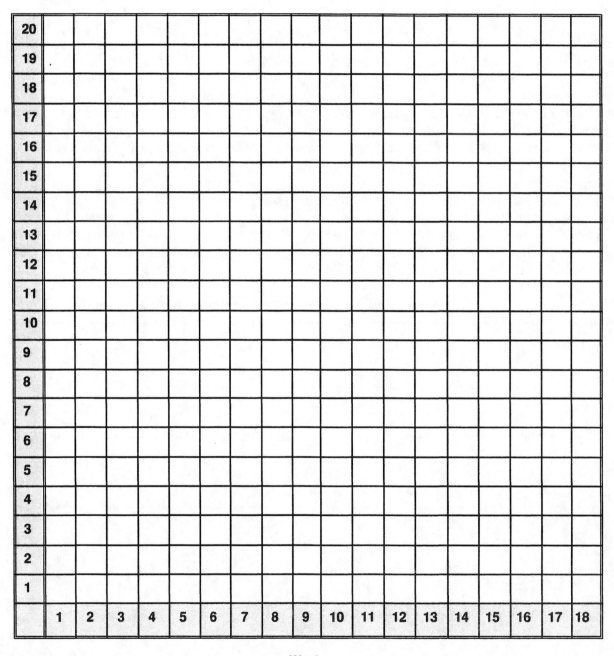

Week

IV

Self-Management and Assertiveness

Weekly Behavior Inventory

Handout

Client name: _____ Date: _____

Please list the approximate number of times you have been involved in the events listed below during the last week. If you were the one slapped, etc., put the number of times. If you did the slapping, etc., put the number of times.

HAPPENED TO ME

Pinching _____
Slapping _____
Grabbing _____
Kicking _____
Punching _____
Hair pulling _____
Throwing things _____
Throwing mate or shoving _____
Hitting with physical object _____
Choking _____
Threat of or use of weapon _____
Burning _____
Sexual abuse _____
Destruction of property _____
Verbal abuse _____
Emotional abuse _____

I DID TO PARTNER

Pinching _____
Slapping _____
Grabbing _____
Kicking _____
Punching _____
Hair pulling _____
Throwing things _____
Throwing mate or shoving _____
Hitting with physical object _____
Choking _____
Threat of or use of weapon _____
Burning _____
Sexual abuse _____
Destruction of property _____
Verbal abuse _____
Emotional abuse _____
Acted assertively _____
Communicated effectively _____
Used time-out _____
Controlled angry behavior _____

I DID HOMEWORK _____

HAPPENED TO CHILDREN

Pinching _____
Slapping _____
Grabbing _____
Hair pulling _____
Kicking _____
Punching _____
Throwing child _____
Hitting with physical object _____
Scarring child _____
Use of weapon _____
Threat of use of weapon _____
Burning _____
Sexual abuse _____
Verbal abuse _____
Emotional abuse _____

I DID TO CHILDREN

Pinching _____
Slapping _____
Grabbing _____
Hair pulling _____
Kicking _____
Punching _____
Throwing child _____
Hitting with physical object _____
Scarring child _____
Use of weapon _____
Threat of use of weapon _____
Burning _____
Sexual abuse _____
Verbal abuse _____
Emotional abuse _____
Acted assertively _____
Communicated effectively _____
Used time-out _____
Controlled angry behavior _____
Spent quality time _____

I DON'T FEEL SAFE
TALKING IN GROUP _____

Self-Esteem Dynamics

Self-esteem is the value we choose to place on ourselves. It is how we view ourselves, not how others view or value us. We tend to perceive, judge, and act in ways consistent with our self-esteem.

TYPES OF SELF-ESTEEM

1. **Positive Self-Esteem**—This is viewing yourself as worthwhile.
2. **Negative Self-Esteem**—This is viewing yourself as worthless or only worthwhile if you accomplish what you think you should. Sometimes people with negative or low self-esteem have an **inferiority complex.** They may have strong and persistent doubts about their competence. They may feel less important, inadequate, or worthless in comparison to others.

SYMPTOMS OF AN INFERIORITY COMPLEX

- Sensitivity to criticism
- Inappropriate response to flattery
- Tendency toward blaming
- Hypercritical attitude
- Feeling of persecution
- Inappropriate feelings about competition
- Tendency toward remoteness, shyness, and timidity

DIFFERENT AREAS OF SELF-CONCEPTS

1. **Identity**—A person's identity involves having direction for his or her life. It involves answering such questions as "Who am I?" and "What's my purpose in life?"
2. **Self-Acceptance**—Self-acceptance involves knowing and accepting the strengths and weaknesses you have and feeling that you are okay.
3. **Self-Satisfaction**—Self-satisfaction involves being satisfied with who you are and where you are on the road of life. Some dissatisfaction is healthy, because it motivates people to strengthen their weaknesses or change their situations.
4. **Moral, Ethical Self**—The moral, ethical self relates to how you feel about yourself in relation to being ethical in dealing with others and in doing what you feel is right or wrong. It could relate to how you feel about your relationship to a superior being such as God.
5. **Physical Self**—The physical self involves how you feel about your physical appearance, your body, and about your health.
6. **Personal Self**—The personal self relates to how you feel you present yourself to others. It could involve the use of gestures, facial expression, and nonverbal expression.
7. **Family Self**—The family self relates to how you feel about yourself in relation to your family, husband, wife, children, or parents. It could involve whether there are problems in the relationship, or whether you feel the "family" likes you or thinks you are okay.
8. **Peer Self**—The peer self relates to how you feel about yourself in relation to those outside your family. This could include friends, fellow employees, or employers.

Self-Esteem Dynamics *(Continued)*

Handout

WHY IS SELF-ESTEEM SO IMPORTANT

1. It determines how we let others treat us.
2. It affects the decisions and choices we make, such as the spouse we choose, the friends we choose, employment, and so on.
3. It affects our academic and career achievement.
4. It affects how motivated we are or how hard we try.

WHICH SIGNIFICANT FACTORS INFLUENCE OUR SELF-ESTEEM?

1. Parents, family
2. Social class, money
3. Intellectual ability
4. Physical appearance, face, body type
5. Job, role
6. Education
7. Physical strength, stamina
8. Sexual prowess

Some of these are areas that are difficult or impossible to make major changes in and often need to be accepted. One's self-esteem need never become entirely dependent on any of these areas, however. Anytime we put ourselves in a situation in which we compare ourselves with others, we may come out feeling inferior. There are always going to be others who are better looking, have more money, own a better car, have a nicer house, have a higher IQ, and so on.

Self-Concept Homework

Make a list of 5 words you would use to describe yourself, and what they mean to you:

Example: Friendly—Because I say hello and smile when I meet new people.

     Descriptive word   What it means to me

1. _____

2. _____

3. _____

4. _____

5. _____

1. What do you think and feel about yourself?

2. Do you like yourself as you are?

Inventory of Strengths and Weaknesses

Handout

List what you consider to be five of your strengths and five of your weaknesses:

Strengths	Weaknesses

1. _____   1. _____

2. _____   2. _____

3. _____   3. _____

4. _____   4. _____

5. _____   5. _____

Which weaknesses can you change and how?

_____

_____

_____

Which weaknesses do you need to accept and why?

_____

_____

_____

Self-Concept Life Graph

On the graph below plot important events, both positive and negative, in your life. Place these events above or below the neutral line and label your age at the time.

Positive
Events
+

Positive
Events
+

Birth _____ Today

–
Negative
Events

–
Negative
Events

How do you feel about the above picture of your life?

Where is the graph going to go from here? Are you in charge of it?

Weekly Behavior Inventory

Handout

Client name: _____ Date: _____

Please list the approximate number of times you have been involved in the events listed below during the last week. If you were the one slapped, etc., put the number of times. If you did the slapping, etc., put the number of times.

HAPPENED TO ME

Pinching ____
Slapping ____
Grabbing ____
Kicking ____
Punching ____
Hair pulling ____
Throwing things ____
Throwing mate or shoving ____
Hitting with physical object ____
Choking ____
Threat of or use of weapon ____
Burning ____
Sexual abuse ____
Destruction of property ____
Verbal abuse ____
Emotional abuse ____

HAPPENED TO CHILDREN

Pinching ____
Slapping ____
Grabbing ____
Hair pulling ____
Kicking ____
Punching ____
Throwing child ____
Hitting with physical object ____
Scarring child ____
Use of weapon ____
Threat of use of weapon ____
Burning ____
Sexual abuse ____
Verbal abuse ____
Emotional abuse ____

I DID TO PARTNER

Pinching ____
Slapping ____
Grabbing ____
Kicking ____
Punching ____
Hair pulling ____
Throwing things ____
Throwing mate or shoving ____
Hitting with physical object ____
Choking ____
Threat of or use of weapon ____
Burning ____
Sexual abuse ____
Destruction of property ____
Verbal abuse ____
Emotional abuse ____
Acted assertively ____
Communicated effectively ____
Used time-out ____
Controlled angry behavior ____

I DID HOMEWORK ____

I DID TO CHILDREN

Pinching ____
Slapping ____
Grabbing ____
Hair pulling ____
Kicking ____
Punching ____
Throwing child ____
Hitting with physical object ____
Scarring child ____
Use of weapon ____
Threat of use of weapon ____
Burning ____
Sexual abuse ____
Verbal abuse ____
Emotional abuse ____
Acted assertively ____
Communicated effectively ____
Used time-out ____
Controlled angry behavior ____
Spent quality time ____

I DON'T FEEL SAFE
TALKING IN GROUP ____

Techniques for Changing Self-Esteem

1. **Rewrite Internal Monologue—The Way You Talk to Yourself**

   A. **Accept the past: You can't change it.** No matter when, where, or how something happened in the past, you cannot go back and change it. What you can do is change the present.

   B. **Quit putting yourself down.** The purpose of life is to find enjoyment and meaning, not to evaluate yourself. Give up "shoulds," "oughts," and "musts," and replace them with "wants."

   Example   Say to yourself, "I want to be the best person at my job." Do not say, "I must be the best person at my job."

   C. **Think about good experiences you have had in the past.** Be proud of your achievements. Dwell on your successes, not your failures. Use the techniques that helped you be successful in the past.

   Example   If you did well in athletics, then get active in some type of sport again.

   D. **Make positive goals for the future.** With small, realistic goals you will be successful and motivated to reach your end goal.

   Example   If you want to lose weight, make a goal to lose a pound a week. Continue to try to do this every week until you reach your desired weight. This is much more realistic than a goal to lose 25 pounds in 1 month.

   E. **Techniques for thought change.**

   - Record negative thoughts in detail. This will help you be aware of the negative thoughts you are having. Also, it will help you discover their patterns and what triggers them. Awareness helps you change and control negative thoughts.
   - Block negative thoughts. When you have a negative thought tell yourself silently or out loud to **STOP**. Refuse to allow yourself to think negatively.
   - Replace negative thoughts with positive thoughts. After saying **"STOP"** to the negative thought, think of a positive thought immediately. Remember to draw from your successes.

2. **Diagnose Lowered Self-Esteem Cues**

   A. **Decide what situations cue low self-esteem.** Do you feel inferior when you think someone is not interested in what you say? (Rejection) Are you comparing yourself to others: physically, intellectually, financially? Is it the circumstance, event, setting, or interpersonal interaction that are making you feel this way? Is it because of physical or personal isolation?

   B. **Use your knowledge of what cues lower self-esteem to help you overcome it.** It may be necessary to avoid certain things or situations that make you feel this way. Or you may choose to work on improving in a certain area.

   Example   If lowered self-esteem is a result of non-assertiveness, then you could attend assertiveness-training classes to improve this skill.

Techniques for Changing Self-Esteem *(Continued)*

3. **Learn to Relax**

   A. **Relaxation.** Lie or sit in a comfortable position. Close your eyes. Breathe deeply, tense and relax each muscle group. Begin with your arm, move on to your abdomen, legs, neck, and facial muscles. Concentrate on feelings of warmth and relaxation. Practice doing this at least once a day. Review Session 4.
   B. **Exercise.** Choose something you like and will continue doing. Join an aerobics class or ride your bike. Pick a time of day that is convenient and exercise at least 2–3 times a week.

4. **Modify Unrealistic Standards**

   A. **Rational thinking.** You are influenced by your view and perception of the world. Often this takes precedence over actual reality. How you see things is often more important than what really happened. Your beliefs about yourself influence how you feel and what you do.

      Example   Your boss tells you that you made a mistake in your last project (event); you tell yourself, "I am worthless" (belief). You become depressed and feel horrible about yourself (emotion).
      The point is that bad things happen. Acknowledge that this is a fact of life. Do not give yourself additional stress by following a belief system that hurts you. Adopt a healthy belief system, and you will be happier and more successful.

   B. **Are your expectations reasonable and obtainable?** Again, set your expectations and goals so that they are obtainable. Do not place obstacles in your way by making goals that demand perfection or that are impossible to reach. Make small goals that lead to your end goal. Reward yourself when you reach each goal.
   C. **Don't expect perfection in yourself or others.** This sets you up for failure. Enjoy your uniqueness and that of others. Learn to appreciate yourself and others. Again, stop rating yourself or others. Give yourself freedom to make mistakes and still like who you are. Extend this freedom to others also.

5. **Create Better Social Support Reinforcement**

   A. **Seek people who give you positive reinforcement.**
   B. **Be pleasant to others.** Talk and act in a positive manner.
   C. **Be nice, even when you do not feel like it.**
   D. **Do not expect everyone to like you.**
   E. **Do not expect everyone to be perfect.**
   F. **Do not talk about your problems all the time.** Others do not like to hear negative things constantly. Think about positive and funny events.
   G. **Be assertive, not aggressive.** Let people know what you want and need in an appropriate way. Do not expect them to know what you need.

Techniques for Changing
Self-Esteem *(Continued)*

6. **Learn to Meet Your Needs**

   A. **Love and be loved.** Giving up unrealistic demands on yourself and others allows you to love and be loved more generously. Having a loving relationship with at least one other person may be crucial to your well-being.

   B. **Feel worthwhile.** Doing something you feel is useful and worthwhile is important for everyone. Give yourself credit for anything you are doing that makes you feel worthwhile.

   C. **Have fun.** Allow yourself to have fun. Do something that you find enjoyable every day. If there is something that is particularly fun to you that you have not done for some time, make it a point to indulge in this activity very soon.

   Example   Have your hair done, have a manicure, go rollerskating, go to a ball game, go bowling, play tennis, or call your best friend from high school.

   D. **Be free.** Keep in mind at all times that you are free to make choices. Forget the past and live in the present. Accept responsibility for making meaningful choices in your life. You are free to choose how to live your life.

Weekly Behavior Inventory

Handout

Client name: _____ Date: _____

Please list the approximate number of times you have been involved in the events listed below during the last week. If you were the one slapped, etc., put the number of times. If you did the slapping, etc., put the number of times.

HAPPENED TO ME

Pinching ____
Slapping ____
Grabbing ____
Kicking ____
Punching ____
Hair pulling ____
Throwing things ____
Throwing mate or shoving ____
Hitting with physical object ____
Choking ____
Threat of or use of weapon ____
Burning ____
Sexual abuse ____
Destruction of property ____
Verbal abuse ____
Emotional abuse ____

HAPPENED TO CHILDREN

Pinching ____
Slapping ____
Grabbing ____
Hair pulling ____
Kicking ____
Punching ____
Throwing child ____
Hitting with physical object ____
Scarring child ____
Use of weapon ____
Threat of use of weapon ____
Burning ____
Sexual abuse ____
Verbal abuse ____
Emotional abuse ____

I DID TO PARTNER

Pinching ____
Slapping ____
Grabbing ____
Kicking ____
Punching ____
Hair pulling ____
Throwing things ____
Throwing mate or shoving ____
Hitting with physical object ____
Choking ____
Threat of or use of weapon ____
Burning ____
Sexual abuse ____
Destruction of property ____
Verbal abuse ____
Emotional abuse ____
Acted assertively ____
Communicated effectively ____
Used time-out ____
Controlled angry behavior ____

I DID HOMEWORK ____

I DID TO CHILDREN

Pinching ____
Slapping ____
Grabbing ____
Hair pulling ____
Kicking ____
Punching ____
Throwing child ____
Hitting with physical object ____
Scarring child ____
Use of weapon ____
Threat of use of weapon ____
Burning ____
Sexual abuse ____
Verbal abuse ____
Emotional abuse ____
Acted assertively ____
Communicated effectively ____
Used time-out ____
Controlled angry behavior ____
Spent quality time ____

I DON'T FEEL SAFE
TALKING IN GROUP ____

Faulty Self-Talk

1. **BLACK & WHITE:** This is the tendency to see things in an all-or-nothing fashion. Beware of words like "never," "always," "nothing," and "everyone."

    "Real men don't eat quiche."
    "You're either on my side or you're not."
    "You can't trust anyone over 30."

2. **MINIMIZING:** This is the tendency to downplay your achievements.

    "Even though I finally got my promotion, it's no big thing."
    "I did well, but so did a lot of other people."
    "My counselor just gives me good feedback because she's paid to say it."

3. **MIND-READING:** This is the tendency to assume that others think something without determining if this is really so.

    "I know my boss hates me . . . he gave me a dirty look."
    "She's avoiding me . . . she must be pretty mad."
    "My husband didn't call me today . . . he must not care about me."

4. **AWFULIZING:** This is the tendency to predict that things will turn out "awful" for you.

    "My brother will never trust me again."
    "I know I'm not going to make it through this place."

5. **ERROR IN BLAMING:** This is the tendency to unfairly blame yourself or others.

    "It's all my fault" or "It's all their fault."
    "It's my fault my son is shy."
    "You always mess everything up for me."

6. **PUT-DOWNS:** This is the tendency to put yourself down for having one problem or making one mistake.

    "I'm overweight, so I must be lazy and stupid."
    "I failed this test, so I must be dumb."
    "I'm in counseling, I must be a bad person."
    "She doesn't like me, I must be ugly."

7. **EMOTIONAL REASONING:** This is the tendency to conclude that if you feel a certain way about yourself, then it must be true.

    "Because I feel bad about myself, I must be a bad person."
    "I feel rejected, so everybody must be rejecting me."
    "Because I feel guilty, I must have done something wrong."

Unproductive Self-Talk

Handout

- She wants to be with someone else.

- If she's out alone, someone will pick her up.

- He never does what I want.

- No one understands.

- If I'm not tough, she'll think I'm weak.

- I need to show her I'm in control.

- If she talks to another man, it means she wants to go to bed with him.

- She does nothing but stay home, take care of the kids, and talk on the phone.

- If other women look at him, it means he is flirting with them, which demeans me.

- She is responsible for other men's reactions to her.

- He's out to make me a fool.

- She keeps the kids from respecting me.

- His wanting time for himself means he doesn't want me.

- His not being there when I want him means he doesn't care.

- I'm sick and tired of all this crap.

- No matter what I do, it won't be good enough.

- The kids are more important to her than I am.

- His family is more important to him than I am.

Adapted from *Battering: AMEND Manual for Helpers*, AMEND Program, Denver, CO.

Weekly Behavior Inventory

Handout

Client name: _____ Date: _____

Please list the approximate number of times you have been involved in the events listed below during the last week. If you were the one slapped, etc., put the number of times. If you did the slapping, etc., put the number of times.

HAPPENED TO ME

Pinching _____
Slapping _____
Grabbing _____
Kicking _____
Punching _____
Hair pulling _____
Throwing things _____
Throwing mate or shoving _____
Hitting with physical object _____
Choking _____
Threat of or use of weapon _____
Burning _____
Sexual abuse _____
Destruction of property _____
Verbal abuse _____
Emotional abuse _____

HAPPENED TO CHILDREN

Pinching _____
Slapping _____
Grabbing _____
Hair pulling _____
Kicking _____
Punching _____
Throwing child _____
Hitting with physical object _____
Scarring child _____
Use of weapon _____
Threat of use of weapon _____
Burning _____
Sexual abuse _____
Verbal abuse _____
Emotional abuse _____

I DID TO PARTNER

Pinching _____
Slapping _____
Grabbing _____
Kicking _____
Punching _____
Hair pulling _____
Throwing things _____
Throwing mate or shoving _____
Hitting with physical object _____
Choking _____
Threat of or use of weapon _____
Burning _____
Sexual abuse _____
Destruction of property _____
Verbal abuse _____
Emotional abuse _____
Acted assertively _____
Communicated effectively _____
Used time-out _____
Controlled angry behavior _____

I DID HOMEWORK _____

I DID TO CHILDREN

Pinching _____
Slapping _____
Grabbing _____
Hair pulling _____
Kicking _____
Punching _____
Throwing child _____
Hitting with physical object _____
Scarring child _____
Use of weapon _____
Threat of use of weapon _____
Burning _____
Sexual abuse _____
Verbal abuse _____
Emotional abuse _____
Acted assertively _____
Communicated effectively _____
Used time-out _____
Controlled angry behavior _____
Spent quality time _____

**I DON'T FEEL SAFE
TALKING IN GROUP** _____

Using Cognitive Reframing

Think of a situation that you responded to emotionally. Follow the six-step method of uncovering, reframing, and changing the distorted situation to restructure your thinking.

Step 1.   **Recognize and label what you were feeling.**

Step 2.   **Describe the situation or experience that led to the emotions.**

Step 3.   **Identify the distorted self-talk or negative perceptions.**

Step 4.   **Rephrase the self-talk to be more positive and rational.**

Step 5.   **Plan behavior based on new self-talk.**

Step 6.   **Recognize and label your emotion after the positive self-talk. What are you feeling now? Reward yourself for coping.**

Example   A wife feels unloved and taken for granted because her husband did not call today.

Step 1.   Recognize feelings of being unloved, lonely, fearful, and angey.

Step 2.   Spouse hasn't called.

Step 3.   Distorted self-talk says that because he hasn't called, he must not love her and doesn't consider her feelings.

Step 4.   Rephrase self-talk by thinking that her spouse must have gotten involved at work and did not have time to call. She should not expect her husband to call every day. It is irrational to base her thoughts of how much her husband cares about her on whether he calls every day or not.

Step 5.   Decide to talk with spouse about taking some time for the two of them to go away together for a few days.

Step 6.   Wife feels more positive about herself and her relationship.

Changing Your Self-Talk

Handout

FOR WOMEN

Category	Faulty Self-Talk	Positive Self-Talk
Fearful and Anxious	I'm afraid I will always be alone.	I can have close relationships with others and I can depend on myself.
Anger and Frustration	There is something wrong with me for being mad—I should not feel this way.	My spouse is responsible for the abuse, and my anger is a normal response.
Guilt and Remorse	I am responsible for the abuse—I caused it.	My partner is responsible for the abuse. I was a victim.
Shame and Self-Disgust	I will always be helpless. I cannot control my life.	I can take control of my life.
Sadness	I am empty.	I am whole and I can be happy. It is up to me.

FOR MEN

Category	Faulty Self-Talk	Positive Self-Talk
Fearful and Anxious	If I don't control her she will leave me.	She is a free person. She is more likely to stay if I do not try to control her.
Anger and Frustration	I don't mean to hurt her, but she makes me do it.	I am in control of myself and I take full responsibility for my behavior.
Guilt and Remorse	She makes me hurt her and then I feel bad.	When I control my actions I feel good about myself.
Shame and Self-Disgust	I am not confident in myself. I cannot trust anyone.	I feel confident in some areas of my life. I trust myself. I can trust some people.
Sadness	I am sad. There is no hope.	I can change. I can be happy. It is up to me.

Weekly Behavior Inventory

Handout

Client name: _____ Date: _____

Please list the approximate number of times you have been involved in the events listed below during the last week. If you were the one slapped, etc., put the number of times. If you did the slapping, etc., put the number of times.

HAPPENED TO ME

Pinching _____
Slapping _____
Grabbing _____
Kicking _____
Punching _____
Hair pulling _____
Throwing things _____
Throwing mate or shoving _____
Hitting with physical object _____
Choking _____
Threat of or use of weapon _____
Burning _____
Sexual abuse _____
Destruction of property _____
Verbal abuse _____
Emotional abuse _____

I DID TO PARTNER

Pinching _____
Slapping _____
Grabbing _____
Kicking _____
Punching _____
Hair pulling _____
Throwing things _____
Throwing mate or shoving _____
Hitting with physical object _____
Choking _____
Threat of or use of weapon _____
Burning _____
Sexual abuse _____
Destruction of property _____
Verbal abuse _____
Emotional abuse _____
Acted assertively _____
Communicated effectively _____
Used time-out _____
Controlled angry behavior _____

I DID HOMEWORK _____

HAPPENED TO CHILDREN

Pinching _____
Slapping _____
Grabbing _____
Hair pulling _____
Kicking _____
Punching _____
Throwing child _____
Hitting with physical object _____
Scarring child _____
Use of weapon _____
Threat of use of weapon _____
Burning _____
Sexual abuse _____
Verbal abuse _____
Emotional abuse _____

I DID TO CHILDREN

Pinching _____
Slapping _____
Grabbing _____
Hair pulling _____
Kicking _____
Punching _____
Throwing child _____
Hitting with physical object _____
Scarring child _____
Use of weapon _____
Threat of use of weapon _____
Burning _____
Sexual abuse _____
Verbal abuse _____
Emotional abuse _____
Acted assertively _____
Communicated effectively _____
Used time-out _____
Controlled angry behavior _____
Spent quality time _____

I DON'T FEEL SAFE
TALKING IN GROUP _____

Counters

☐ These thoughts are unproductive and harmful.

☐ I trust her.

☐ She hasn't given me any reason not to trust her.

☐ He may be right.

☐ I can be assertive.

☐ I can take a time-out.

☐ I'm important to her even though it may not seem that way now.

☐ I'm in control.

☐ She/he/they can't get me upset unless I allow them to.

☐ It's too nice of a day to get upset.

☐ I need to do something for myself that's relaxing.

☐ It's okay that she's angry, I don't have to settle it right now.

☐ I can say no.

☐ I can negotiate and offer a compromise.

☐ I can ask for what I want.

Taken from *Battering: AMEND Manual for Helpers*, AMEND Program, 1984, Denver, CO.

Coping Plan for Stressor Situations

Handout

If you believe that you are being frustrated, annoyed, insulted, or attacked and begin to feel angry:

1. Don't respond immediately.
2. Take several short deep breaths to fill your chest and relax as you breathe out.
3. Think of other possible explanations for what is making you angry.
4. Think of the consequences of reacting in different ways.
5. Start to respond in some way that will control your anger and would be an alternative to aggression.

STRESS INOCULATION FOR ANGER CONTROL: COMMON COPING STATEMENTS FOR STRESSOR SITUATIONS

1. **Prepare for Stressful Situations**
   This could be a rough situation, but I know how to deal with it. I can work out a plan to handle this. Easy does it. Remember, stick to the issues and don't take it personally. There won't be any need for an argument. I know what to do.

2. **Meeting the Situation**
   As long as I keep my cool, I'm in control of the situation. I don't need to prove myself. Don't make more of this than I have to. There is no point in getting mad. Think of what I have to do. Look for the positive and do not jump to conclusions.

3. **Coping with Arousal**
   My muscles are getting tight; relax and slow things down. Time to take a deep breath. Let's take the issue point by point. My anger is a signal of what I need to do. Time for problem solving. He or she probably wants me to get angry, but I'm going to deal with it constructively.

4. **Subsequent Reflection**
   Conflict Unresolved—Forget about the mistakes now. Thinking about it only makes me upset. Try to shake it off. Do not let it interfere with my job. Remember relaxation; it is a lot better than anger. Do not take it personally. It may not be so serious.
   Conflict Resolved—I handled that one pretty well. That means I'm doing a good job. I could have gotten more upset than it was worth. My pride can get me into trouble, but I am doing better at this all the time. I actually got through this without getting angry.

Adapted from Raymond Novaco, 1979.

Weekly Behavior Inventory

Handout

Client name: _____ Date: _____

Please list the approximate number of times you have been involved in the events listed below during the last week. If you were the one slapped, etc., put the number of times. If you did the slapping, etc., put the number of times.

HAPPENED TO ME

Pinching _____
Slapping _____
Grabbing _____
Kicking _____
Punching _____
Hair pulling _____
Throwing things _____
Throwing mate or shoving _____
Hitting with physical object _____
Choking _____
Threat of or use of weapon _____
Burning _____
Sexual abuse _____
Destruction of property _____
Verbal abuse _____
Emotional abuse _____

I DID TO PARTNER

Pinching _____
Slapping _____
Grabbing _____
Kicking _____
Punching _____
Hair pulling _____
Throwing things _____
Throwing mate or shoving _____
Hitting with physical object _____
Choking _____
Threat of or use of weapon _____
Burning _____
Sexual abuse _____
Destruction of property _____
Verbal abuse _____
Emotional abuse _____
Acted assertively _____
Communicated effectively _____
Used time-out _____
Controlled angry behavior _____

I DID HOMEWORK _____

HAPPENED TO CHILDREN

Pinching _____
Slapping _____
Grabbing _____
Hair pulling _____
Kicking _____
Punching _____
Throwing child _____
Hitting with physical object _____
Scarring child _____
Use of weapon _____
Threat of use of weapon _____
Burning _____
Sexual abuse _____
Verbal abuse _____
Emotional abuse _____

I DID TO CHILDREN

Pinching _____
Slapping _____
Grabbing _____
Hair pulling _____
Kicking _____
Punching _____
Throwing child _____
Hitting with physical object _____
Scarring child _____
Use of weapon _____
Threat of use of weapon _____
Burning _____
Sexual abuse _____
Verbal abuse _____
Emotional abuse _____
Acted assertively _____
Communicated effectively _____
Used time-out _____
Controlled angry behavior _____
Spent quality time _____

I DON'T FEEL SAFE TALKING IN GROUP _____

Dynamics of Assertiveness

TYPES OF BEHAVIOR

1. **Assertive**   This behavior involves knowing what you feel and want. It also involves expressing your feelings and wants directly and honestly without violating the rights of others. At all times you are accepting responsibility for your feelings and actions.

> Example: A person goes to the store and buys a blouse. There is a seam undone. He or she takes it back to the store and asks in a friendly but firm manner for a new blouse or a refund.

2. **Aggressive**   This type of behavior involves attacking others, being controlling, provoking, and maybe even violent. Its consequences could be harmful to others as well as yourself.

> Example: Consider the same situation as the one above. The person takes the blouse back to the store and yells at the salesclerk and acts in a demanding manner.

3. **Passive**   With this behavior, the person has the tendency to withdraw, become anxious, and avoid confrontation. Passive people let others think for them, make decisions for them, and tell them what to do. Many times this causes the person to feel hurt, depressed, and lowers their self-esteem.

> Example: Again, consider the same blouse scenario. The customer gets angry but does not express or deal with the anger. Depression will likely follow, he or she may believe that the salesperson sold the blouse to him or her on purpose, but does nothing about the situation.

4. **Passive-Aggressive**   With this behavior, the person is not direct in relating to people, does not accept what is happening, but will retaliate in an indirect manner. This type of behavior can cause extensive confusion because no one knows what the real issues are.

> Example: When confronted with the poorly sewn blouse, the passive-aggressive person will say bad things about the store to others, mess up the merchandise on the shelves, and so on. The person never directly approaches any solution or confronts the problem, however.

What Is Assertive Behavior?

Handout

- Asking for what you want but not being demanding.
- Being able to express feelings.
- Being able to genuinely express feedback or compliments to others and being able to accept them.
- Being able to disagree without being aggressive.
- Being able to use "I" messages and "I feel" statements without being judgmental or blaming.
- Avoiding arguing just for the sake of arguing.
- Making eye contact during a conversation.

SUMMARY

Assertiveness is a way of communicating in which we make our needs, feelings, thoughts, and desires known without decreasing our rights and self-esteem, nor the rights and self-esteem of others.

Examples:

1. Honey, could we go out to eat? I'm sure tired from my day.
2. I feel embarrassed when you tease me about my weight in front of my friends.
3. I'm sorry you didn't enjoy the evening; I thought it was a lot of fun.
4. Susie, I'm having some difficulty disciplining Joey; could you give me some pointers?
5. Jerry, I feel angry when you are late and don't call.
6. Sara, could we talk about this after we've both cooled off?
7. Look the person in the eye and say, "I really care about you, let's work this out."

Benefits of Assertiveness

Handout

What benefits are there for being more assertive?

- I can be more independent.
- I can make my own decisions.
- I can have more open and honest relationships.
- Others will respect my rights and wishes.
- I can take control of my own emotions.
- I can be more relaxed and at peace with myself.
- I can get satisfaction in initiating and carrying out my own plans.
- I can get more of what I need and want.

Situations and Behaviors

Keep a record of different interpersonal situations that occur during the week. Record what your body cues were, whether your behavior was assertive, aggressive, passive, or passive/aggressive. Record how you felt. Decide if you feel good about how you responded. If not, record what you would like to have done and why you didn't do it.

Situation and date	Physical body cues	How I felt	My behavior (As., Ag., P., P-Ag.)	What I would like to have done	Why I did not do it

Weekly Behavior Inventory

Handout

Client name: _____   Date: _____

Please list the approximate number of times you have been involved in the events listed below during the last week. If you were the one slapped, etc., put the number of times. If you did the slapping, etc., put the number of times.

HAPPENED TO ME

Pinching	____
Slapping	____
Grabbing	____
Kicking	____
Punching	____
Hair pulling	____
Throwing things	____
Throwing mate or shoving	____
Hitting with physical object	____
Choking	____
Threat of or use of weapon	____
Burning	____
Sexual abuse	____
Destruction of property	____
Verbal abuse	____
Emotional abuse	____

HAPPENED TO CHILDREN

Pinching	____
Slapping	____
Grabbing	____
Hair pulling	____
Kicking	____
Punching	____
Throwing child	____
Hitting with physical object	____
Scarring child	____
Use of weapon	____
Threat of use of weapon	____
Burning	____
Sexual abuse	____
Verbal abuse	____
Emotional abuse	____

I DID TO PARTNER

Pinching	____
Slapping	____
Grabbing	____
Kicking	____
Punching	____
Hair pulling	____
Throwing things	____
Throwing mate or shoving	____
Hitting with physical object	____
Choking	____
Threat of or use of weapon	____
Burning	____
Sexual abuse	____
Destruction of property	____
Verbal abuse	____
Emotional abuse	____
Acted assertively	____
Communicated effectively	____
Used time-out	____
Controlled angry behavior	____

I DID TO CHILDREN

Pinching	____
Slapping	____
Grabbing	____
Hair pulling	____
Kicking	____
Punching	____
Throwing child	____
Hitting with physical object	____
Scarring child	____
Use of weapon	____
Threat of use of weapon	____
Burning	____
Sexual abuse	____
Verbal abuse	____
Emotional abuse	____
Acted assertively	____
Communicated effectively	____
Used time-out	____
Controlled angry behavior	____
Spent quality time	____

I DID HOMEWORK ____

I DON'T FEEL SAFE TALKING IN GROUP ____

Tips on Assertiveness

- Begin statements with the pronoun "I," such as "I feel hurt when . . ."

- Do not feel that you have to justify, rationalize, or give reasons for how you feel.

- Move closer to the person with whom you are talking.

- When you do not want to do something, say "no," and do not feel that you have to apologize or make excuses. Learn to say "no" many different ways, firmly and graciously.

- Be responsible to yourself first in getting your needs met, but without attacking other's rights. You do not have to be perfect or prove how "nice" you are.

- Remember it's costly not to be assertive.

- Sometimes you may need to persist in being assertive until others realize what you want.

Learning to Say "No"

Handout

Possible reasons you say "yes" when you want to say "no."

- You want to be liked or accepted.
- It makes you feel you are a good person for helping others.
- You don't want to hurt anyone's feelings.
- What would the family think?
- You want the other person to feel obliged.

You have a right to say "no."

- When your priorities do not go along with the request.
- When the person can do it him or herself.
- When it's against your values and judgments.
- If you would feel bad doing it.
- If it would hurt you or someone else.
- If the demand is inappropriate.
- If you just don't want to do it.
- If the request is inconsiderate of you or others.

Compliments

Assertive people know how to sincerely give compliments as well as receive them.

WHAT WE COMPLIMENT

- Behavior—I appreciate you being so **attentive** when I'm feeling ill.
- Appearance—You really **look good** in that bathing suit.
- Possessions—That's a **nice tie.**

THE GOLDEN RULE

Give more compliments than criticism, more praise than punishment.

Delivery

- Be specific.
- Use the other person's name.
- Add an explanatory sentence.
- Personalize the compliment.
- Ask a question.
- Practice good nonverbal communication.

   Example: Ethel, I like the way you take the time in getting the children involved in activities.

Other ways to compliment

- **The third-person compliment:** Compliment the person within earshot or tell someone you know will repeat the compliment directly to the person.
- **The relayed compliment:** Pass on a compliment from another person; follow with an example.
- **The indirect compliment:** Words and actions can signal admiration; ask for the person's opinion or advice.
- **The nonverbal compliment:** Smiles, nods, eye contact, and other positive body language can be complimentary.

COMPLIMENT GUIDELINES

- Be honest.
- Start slowly.
- Be conservative at first.
- Avoid the hidden agenda.
- Do not repeat the exact same compliment.
- Favorably compare the person to others.
- Do not get carried away.
- Avoid being Mr./Mrs. Positive.

Compliments *(Continued)*

Handout

HOW TO ACCEPT A COMPLIMENT

- Make eye contact.
- Assume an open posture.
- Smile.
- Thank the other person.
- Use the other person's name.
- Give credit if appropriate.
- Tell the other person how you feel about the compliment.
- Self-disclose.

  Remember:
- Never discount a compliment.
- Do not return the same compliment unless appropriate.

Asking for What You Want

Handout

What are the advantages of asking for what you want? We hope the first thing you thought of was increasing the chances of getting what you want in life. Though there is no guarantee you will always get your way, the odds are more in your favor than if you do not ask, and instead expect others to read your mind. Just as with yourself, the person of whom we are making the request has the right to say no, with or without an explanation. With this in mind, let's begin by giving you some practice in asking for what you want.

ASKING FOR WHAT YOU WANT

Place two chairs facing each other. You sit in one and have your partner sit in the other. Make the following requests out loud and see how it feels to ask these questions. Are there any areas that feel more or less comfortable? Rate the difficulty of each request on a 1 to 5 scale (1 being easy and 5 being difficult). Explain why some were more difficult.

_____   1. I would like to borrow $5.00 from you.
_____   2. Would you be willing to help me clean the garage today?
_____   3. I would like to be alone today.
_____   4. I would like to have sex with you.
_____   5. I would like to borrow $100.00.
_____   6. Will you hold me? I'm feeling scared.
_____   7. Will you sleep close to me tonight?
_____   8. I would like to sleep alone tonight.
_____   9. I would like a date with you on Friday.
_____ 10. I would like to talk quietly.
_____ 11. Will you kiss me?
_____ 12. I would like to know why you are angry with me.
_____ 13. Will you take care of the kids today?
_____ 14. How are you feeling today?
_____ 15. I would like to read the paper; can we talk later?
_____ 16. I would like to take a time-out.

ASKING FOR WHAT YOU WANT—HOMEWORK

Asking for what you want would be easier if you begin to make requests of people with whom you are comfortable or at least somewhat comfortable asserting yourself with. Choose a couple of people who you categorized as **comfortable** and **somewhat uncomfortable** to make your requests of this week. Make three requests this week. Indicate the request, how it felt, and how you could improve the way in which you expressed it. Were you direct or in direct (escalating and/or stuffing)? Be sure to use an "I" statement followed by a clear request. Use the examples presented earlier as a guide for how to make your request.

Adapted from Sonkin and Durphy (1989). *Learning to Live Without Violence*. Volcano, CA: Volcano Press. Reprinted by permission of Volcano Press.

V

Intimacy Issues and
Relapse Prevention

Weekly Behavior Inventory

Handout

Client name: _____   Date: _____

Please list the approximate number of times you have been involved in the events listed below during the last week. If you were the one slapped, etc., put the number of times. If you did the slapping, etc., put the number of times.

HAPPENED TO ME

Pinching ____
Slapping ____
Grabbing ____
Kicking ____
Punching ____
Hair pulling ____
Throwing things ____
Throwing mate or shoving ____
Hitting with physical object ____
Choking ____
Threat of or use of weapon ____
Burning ____
Sexual abuse ____
Destruction of property ____
Verbal abuse ____
Emotional abuse ____

HAPPENED TO CHILDREN

Pinching ____
Slapping ____
Grabbing ____
Hair pulling ____
Kicking ____
Punching ____
Throwing child ____
Hitting with physical object ____
Scarring child ____
Use of weapon ____
Threat of use of weapon ____
Burning ____
Sexual abuse ____
Verbal abuse ____
Emotional abuse ____

I DID TO PARTNER

Pinching ____
Slapping ____
Grabbing ____
Kicking ____
Punching ____
Hair pulling ____
Throwing things ____
Throwing mate or shoving ____
Hitting with physical object ____
Choking ____
Threat of or use of weapon ____
Burning ____
Sexual abuse ____
Destruction of property ____
Verbal abuse ____
Emotional abuse ____
Acted assertively ____
Communicated effectively ____
Used time-out ____
Controlled angry behavior ____

I DID HOMEWORK ____

I DID TO CHILDREN

Pinching ____
Slapping ____
Grabbing ____
Hair pulling ____
Kicking ____
Punching ____
Throwing child ____
Hitting with physical object ____
Scarring child ____
Use of weapon ____
Threat of use of weapon ____
Burning ____
Sexual abuse ____
Verbal abuse ____
Emotional abuse ____
Acted assertively ____
Communicated effectively ____
Used time-out ____
Controlled angry behavior ____
Spent quality time ____

**I DON'T FEEL SAFE
    TALKING IN GROUP** ____

Problem Solving

1. **Decide specifically what the problem is.**

   - Do not cast blame.
   - Use "I" messages to express your needs.
   - Verbalize the needs of others involved.
   - Listen to others' view of the problem.
   - Make sure everyone agrees on the definition of the problem.

2. **Brainstorm for possible solutions.**

   - Get possible solutions from others involved.
   - Don't evaluate or discount any solutions at this point.
   - Write down all suggested solutions.

3. **Look at the pros and cons of each possible solution.**

   - Everyone must be honest.
   - Do a lot of critical thinking about possible solutions.

4. **Decide on a solution acceptable to all.**

   - Do not push a solution on others.
   - State the solution so all will be sure they understand.
   - Write down the solution so you can check it later to make sure that it is what each agreed on.

5. **Put the solution into action.**

   - Talk about who will do what and when.
   - Trust each to carry out his or her part.
   - Promote individual responsibility by avoiding reminders, nagging, or monitoring.
   - If someone is not responsible, he or she needs to be confronted using "I" messages.

6. **Evaluate the solution.**

   - Modify the solution if necessary.
   - Check out each person's feelings about the solution.
   - If after a fair amount of time the solution is not working, try another mutually agreed on solution.

Some of the best techniques for problem solving are as follows:

- **Listen actively.**
- **Express feelings honestly.**
- **Care about the needs of others.**
- **Be open to change and revision of solutions if needed.**

Weekly Behavior Inventory

Handout

Client name: _____ Date: _____

Please list the approximate number of times you have been involved in the events listed below during the last week. If you were the one slapped, etc., put the number of times. If you did the slapping, etc., put the number of times.

HAPPENED TO ME

Pinching _____
Slapping _____
Grabbing _____
Kicking _____
Punching _____
Hair pulling _____
Throwing things _____
Throwing mate or shoving _____
Hitting with physical object _____
Choking _____
Threat of or use of weapon _____
Burning _____
Sexual abuse _____
Destruction of property _____
Verbal abuse _____
Emotional abuse _____

I DID TO PARTNER

Pinching _____
Slapping _____
Grabbing _____
Kicking _____
Punching _____
Hair pulling _____
Throwing things _____
Throwing mate or shoving _____
Hitting with physical object _____
Choking _____
Threat of or use of weapon _____
Burning _____
Sexual abuse _____
Destruction of property _____
Verbal abuse _____
Emotional abuse _____
Acted assertively _____
Communicated effectively _____
Used time-out _____
Controlled angry behavior _____

I DID HOMEWORK _____

HAPPENED TO CHILDREN

Pinching _____
Slapping _____
Grabbing _____
Hair pulling _____
Kicking _____
Punching _____
Throwing child _____
Hitting with physical object _____
Scarring child _____
Use of weapon _____
Threat of use of weapon _____
Burning _____
Sexual abuse _____
Verbal abuse _____
Emotional abuse _____

I DID TO CHILDREN

Pinching _____
Slapping _____
Grabbing _____
Hair pulling _____
Kicking _____
Punching _____
Throwing child _____
Hitting with physical object _____
Scarring child _____
Use of weapon _____
Threat of use of weapon _____
Burning _____
Sexual abuse _____
Verbal abuse _____
Emotional abuse _____
Acted assertively _____
Communicated effectively _____
Used time-out _____
Controlled angry behavior _____
Spent quality time _____

I DON'T FEEL SAFE
TALKING IN GROUP _____

Power-and-Control Wheel

PHYSICAL ABUSE

twisting arms, tripping, biting • *pushing, shoving, hitting* • *slapping, choking, pulling hair* • *punching, kicking, grabbing* • *using a weapon against her* • *beating, throwing her down*

POWER AND CONTROL

ISOLATION
Controlling what she does, who she sees and talks to, where she goes.

EMOTIONAL ABUSE
Putting partner down or making them feel bad about themselves. Calling partner names. Making partner think they are crazy. Mind games.

INTIMIDATION
Putting her in fear by: using looks, actions, gestures, loud voice, smashing things.

ECONOMIC ABUSE
Trying to keep her from getting or keeping a job. Making her ask for money, giving her an allowance, taking her money.

USING MALE PRIVILEGE
Treating her like a servant. Making all the "big" decisions. Acting like the "master of the castle."

SEXUAL ABUSE
Making her do sexual things against her will. Physically attacking the sexual parts of her body. Treating her like a sex object.

THREATS
Making and/or carrying out threats to do something to hurt partner emotionally. Threaten to take the children, commit suicide, report partner to welfare.

USING CHILDREN
Making partner feel guilty about the children. Using the children to give messages, using visitation as a way to harass partners.

PHYSICAL ABUSE

Adapted from Domestic Abuse, Intervention Project; Duluth, MN.

Weekly Behavior Inventory

Handout

Client name: _____ Date: _____

Please list the approximate number of times you have been involved in the events listed below during the last week. If you were the one slapped, etc., put the number of times. If you did the slapping, etc., put the number of times.

HAPPENED TO ME

Pinching _____
Slapping _____
Grabbing _____
Kicking _____
Punching _____
Hair pulling _____
Throwing things _____
Throwing mate or shoving _____
Hitting with physical object _____
Choking _____
Threat of or use of weapon _____
Burning _____
Sexual abuse _____
Destruction of property _____
Verbal abuse _____
Emotional abuse _____

HAPPENED TO CHILDREN

Pinching _____
Slapping _____
Grabbing _____
Hair pulling _____
Kicking _____
Punching _____
Throwing child _____
Hitting with physical object _____
Scarring child _____
Use of weapon _____
Threat of use of weapon _____
Burning _____
Sexual abuse _____
Verbal abuse _____
Emotional abuse _____

I DID TO PARTNER

Pinching _____
Slapping _____
Grabbing _____
Kicking _____
Punching _____
Hair pulling _____
Throwing things _____
Throwing mate or shoving _____
Hitting with physical object _____
Choking _____
Threat of or use of weapon _____
Burning _____
Sexual abuse _____
Destruction of property _____
Verbal abuse _____
Emotional abuse _____
Acted assertively _____
Communicated effectively _____
Used time-out _____
Controlled angry behavior _____

I DID HOMEWORK _____

I DID TO CHILDREN

Pinching _____
Slapping _____
Grabbing _____
Hair pulling _____
Kicking _____
Punching _____
Throwing child _____
Hitting with physical object _____
Scarring child _____
Use of weapon _____
Threat of use of weapon _____
Burning _____
Sexual abuse _____
Verbal abuse _____
Emotional abuse _____
Acted assertively _____
Communicated effectively _____
Used time-out _____
Controlled angry behavior _____
Spent quality time _____

I DON'T FEEL SAFE
TALKING IN GROUP _____

Intimacy and Love

How did you get together anyway?

Why were you attracted to each other?

- **Physical Proximity**—Being together, familiarity.

- **Rewards—Anything That Satisfies A Need**—The person may treat you nicely. The benefits and reinforcement of meeting personal needs outweighs the costs.

- **Similarity**—Like backgrounds, interests, attitudes. We assume that others who are similar to us will like us. Similar others often validate our opinions or actions.

- **Opposites**—Sometimes we are attracted to opposites because they provide important needs. Sometimes the very attribute we find attractive initially is what bothers us the most later in the relationship.

    Example: She may feel that he is so strong and a real leader. After they are together for a while, she may view him as domineering and demanding.

- **Doing for Others**—Cognitive dissonance: We like someone for whom we have done a favor.

- **Physical Attractiveness**—Drawn together because of body chemistry or sexual attraction. Sometimes people confuse sexual attraction with love.

- **Self-Esteem**—Sometimes we choose less desirable people because we do not feel we deserve or can get better, or because we may want to feel superior.

STAGES IN RELATIONSHIP DEVELOPMENT

- **Sampling**—This stage involves looking over the possibilities then predicting how satisfying a relationship with this person might be.

- **Bargaining**—This stage involves negotiating mutually satisfying ways of interacting. The couple is trying to get to know each other better and trying to create a way of being together.

- **Commitment**—This stage involves making a mutual decision to spend time together as exclusive partners. This stage is more intimate.

- **Institutionalization**—This is an extension of the commitment stage. It involves some formalization of the commitment (such as marriage). This formalization varies according to cultures and individuals.

PITFALLS IN LOVE RELATIONSHIPS

Pitfalls are common problems that make it difficult to sustain love.

Intimacy and Love *(Continued)*

Handout

BEHAVIOR AT THE BEGINNING OF THE RELATIONSHIP

Individuals may present an idealized self, putting his or her "best foot forward." Other individuals may take the opposite view, however, thinking if the other person can accept his or her worst side, this will be really true love.

The individual may not know him or herself very well and may not accurately perceive the other person.

The individual may mistake sexual attraction for love and find out later they do no even like each other. Society has always glorified romantic love. This involves being wildly excited, sexually aroused, living in a fantasy, and idealizing the relationship. This type of relationship may not be very realistic or enduring.

WHAT IS LOVE?

- **Caring**—This is the feeling that the other person's well-being and satisfaction are as important as your own.

- **Attachment**—This is the need and desire to be with the other person. You want to be approved of and loved by the other person. This does not mean you are dependent on the person.

- **Intimacy**—This involves having close confidential communication and romantic love with its physiological arousal component. Intimacy involves expressing deep feelings, sharing about one's self, and showing tenderness through touching and communicating. Sexual intimacy is also a part of this.

WHAT IS INTIMACY?

Intimacy requires the freedom to be yourself without fear of rejection. It means acceptance without requirements. It is supportive rather than restrictive and combines closeness, trust, and genuine emotion, not possessiveness or control. One must have open, two-way communication, as well as tenderness, affection, warmth, and touching.

A MYTH ABOUT INTIMACY

People often believe that once you find your "one and only," you do not need anyone else. This is not true. No one person can meet all of a person's needs. It is an unrealistic and overwhelming responsibility for one person to have to be "all things" at all times. This is one of the many romantic myths we often fall prey to. We have to work at avoiding these myths.

Eric Fromm, a well-known psychologist, believes that a person's strongest need is love. We need people to listen to us, care about us, and be with us. He sees overcoming isolation and building strong relationships as one of the major tasks of life.

Intimacy and Love *(Continued)*

Handout

HOW CAN WE DEVELOP LOVE OR A LOVING RELATIONSHIP?

Learn all you can about each other. Learn to understand each other's needs. Accept each other as individuals with different needs and desires. Give the relationship time to grow slowly and constantly. Nurture more, criticize less. No one person can meet all of your needs. Give lots of positive attention to each other. Learn to love yourself, so you can love your mate more. It is okay to feel that you are **WONDERFUL!** Learn to express your needs, desires, wants, and feelings. Let your mate express his or her needs, desires, wants, and feelings.

> The act of Love
> is to say,
> "I want you to be
> who you are."
> The act of abuse
> is to say,
> "I want you to be
> who I want
> you to be."
> It is
> that simple.
>
> —James D. Gill

Intimacy Assignment

Handout

What qualities do I want in an intimate relationship?

What qualities can I contribute to an intimate relationship?

Ask your partner what qualities you bring to the relationship. List them below. How do they compare to those you listed above?

Understanding how you express feelings that create intimacy or diminish it helps toward changing or enhancing those expressions. Take a look at the feelings below and state how you express them.

Jealousy _____

Affection _____

Disagreement _____

Rejection _____

Hurt _____

Respect _____

Approval _____

Admiration _____

Anger _____

Love _____

Pride _____

Distress _____

List four people who love you, and beside each name list specific needs that each meets for you.

PEOPLE WHO LOVE ME   **NEEDS THEY MEET**

1. _____   1. _____

2. _____   2. _____

3. _____   3. _____

4. _____   4. _____

Intimacy Assignment *(Continued)*

Handout

There is a lot more to love than just "falling in," and being in love requires energy and a commitment to work for the relationship. Love, like a plant, needs nurturing to grow. What four actions can you take to nurture and help your love relationship grow?

1. _____

2. _____

3. _____

4. _____

Equality Wheel: Nonthreatening Behavior

Handout

NON-VIOLENCE

NEGOTIATION AND FAIRNESS
Seeking mutually satisfying resolutions to conflict. Accepting change. Being willing to compromise

NON-THREATENING BEHAVIOR
Talking and acting so that s/he feels safe and comfortable expressing her/himself and doing things.

ECONOMIC PARTNERSHIP
Making money decisions together. Making sure both partners benefit from financial arrangements.

RESPECT
Listening non-judgmentally. Being emotionally affirming and understanding. Valuing opinions.

EQUALITY

SHARED RESPONSIBILITY
Mutually agreeing on a fair distribution of work. Making family decisions together.

TRUST & SUPPORT
Supporting partner's goals in life. Respecting their right to their own feelings, friends, activities and opinions.

RESPONSIBLE PARENTING
Sharing parental responsibilities. Being a positive non-violent role model for the children.

HONESTY & ACCOUNTABILITY
Accepting responsibility for self. Acknowledging past use of violence. Admitting being wrong. Communicating openly and truthfully.

NON-VIOLENCE

Adapted from: "Tactics of Men Who Batter," Domestic Abuse Intervention Project, Duluth, MN.

© 1999 Springer Publishing Company.

Weekly Behavior Inventory

Client name: _____ Date: _____

Please list the approximate number of times you have been involved in the events listed below during the last week. If you were the one slapped, etc., put the number of times. If you did the slapping, etc., put the number of times.

HAPPENED TO ME

Pinching _____
Slapping _____
Grabbing _____
Kicking _____
Punching _____
Hair pulling _____
Throwing things _____
Throwing mate or shoving _____
Hitting with physical object _____
Choking _____
Threat of or use of weapon _____
Burning _____
Sexual abuse _____
Destruction of property _____
Verbal abuse _____
Emotional abuse _____

HAPPENED TO CHILDREN

Pinching _____
Slapping _____
Grabbing _____
Hair pulling _____
Kicking _____
Punching _____
Throwing child _____
Hitting with physical object _____
Scarring child _____
Use of weapon _____
Threat of use of weapon _____
Burning _____
Sexual abuse _____
Verbal abuse _____
Emotional abuse _____

I DID TO PARTNER

Pinching _____
Slapping _____
Grabbing _____
Kicking _____
Punching _____
Hair pulling _____
Throwing things _____
Throwing mate or shoving _____
Hitting with physical object _____
Choking _____
Threat of or use of weapon _____
Burning _____
Sexual abuse _____
Destruction of property _____
Verbal abuse _____
Emotional abuse _____
Acted assertively _____
Communicated effectively _____
Used time-out _____
Controlled angry behavior _____

I DID TO CHILDREN

Pinching _____
Slapping _____
Grabbing _____
Hair pulling _____
Kicking _____
Punching _____
Throwing child _____
Hitting with physical object _____
Scarring child _____
Use of weapon _____
Threat of use of weapon _____
Burning _____
Sexual abuse _____
Verbal abuse _____
Emotional abuse _____
Acted assertively _____
Communicated effectively _____
Used time-out _____
Controlled angry behavior _____
Spent quality time _____

I DID HOMEWORK _____

I DON'T FEEL SAFE TALKING IN GROUP

Relapse-Prevention Plan

Purpose   To prepare you for future situations when you might be tempted to lose control over your behavior and become aggressive.

Technique   Exposure to "cues" or danger signals that are very likely to lead you toward these behaviors—without letting yourself actually do them. These "cues" can be listed below and then acted out or imagined through visualization.

Cue   1._____

        2._____

        3._____

COPING STRATEGIES

1. **Scare yourself/Support yourself**

    a. Remember how you felt after you blew up, or remember the damage to your family.
    b. After this remembrance, focus on a positive image, such as visualizing yourself in a beautiful place and how you feel when you are able to control your reactions.

2. **Relaxation techniques**

3. **Fun**—Plan to participate in another activity that feels good whenever you notice the old urges, such as physical exercises, listening to music, and so on.

4. **Self-Talk**—Talk to yourself. Call on your supportive observer to help you. What could you say to yourself to help?

5. **Talk to a friend**—Call a friend, therapist, sponsor, crisis center, or family member who can help you cope.

Behavior I Am Trying to Manage: _____

Date _____   Name _____

Adapted from Wexler (1991).

Weekly Behavior Inventory

Handout

Client name: _____   Date: _____

Please list the approximate number of times you have been involved in the events listed below during the last week. If you were the one slapped, etc., put the number of times. If you did the slapping, etc., put the number of times.

HAPPENED TO ME		HAPPENED TO CHILDREN	
Pinching	___	Pinching	___
Slapping	___	Slapping	___
Grabbing	___	Grabbing	___
Kicking	___	Hair pulling	___
Punching	___	Kicking	___
Hair pulling	___	Punching	___
Throwing things	___	Throwing child	___
Throwing mate or shoving	___	Hitting with physical object	___
Hitting with physical object	___	Scarring child	___
Choking	___	Use of weapon	___
Threat of or use of weapon	___	Threat of use of weapon	___
Burning	___	Burning	___
Sexual abuse	___	Sexual abuse	___
Destruction of property	___	Verbal abuse	___
Verbal abuse	___	Emotional abuse	___
Emotional abuse	___		

I DID TO PARTNER		I DID TO CHILDREN	
Pinching	___	Pinching	___
Slapping	___	Slapping	___
Grabbing	___	Grabbing	___
Kicking	___	Hair pulling	___
Punching	___	Kicking	___
Hair pulling	___	Punching	___
Throwing things	___	Throwing child	___
Throwing mate or shoving	___	Hitting with physical object	___
Hitting with physical object	___	Scarring child	___
Choking	___	Use of weapon	___
Threat of or use of weapon	___	Threat of use of weapon	___
Burning	___	Burning	___
Sexual abuse	___	Sexual abuse	___
Destruction of property	___	Verbal abuse	___
Verbal abuse	___	Emotional abuse	___
Emotional abuse	___	Acted assertively	___
Acted assertively	___	Communicated effectively	___
Communicated effectively	___	Used time-out	___
Used time-out	___	Controlled angry behavior	___
Controlled angry behavior	___	Spent quality time	___

I DID HOMEWORK ___

I DON'T FEEL SAFE TALKING IN GROUP ___

Transfer of Change

Handout

Transfer-of-change techniques help you learn to apply what you have learned in group therapy to problem situations outside of group therapy. Actually, we have already used many of the techniques you are now familiar with. Without transfer of change, what you learned in the group would have been perhaps only an interesting exercise that has **no** application to your life.

Maintenance-of-change techniques helps you preserve the level of positive gains you have made in the group. The aim is to make the skills you have learned in the group have a lasting benefit after the group is completed. Sometimes people find it hard to keep their newly learned skills sharp without an active plan for maintaining those skills.

STEPS

Keeping the skills you have learned sharp, improving your performance, and applying what you have learned in the group to other situations takes work, but it is important. The following steps can lead you to a follow-up plan:

1. Become familiar with techniques available to you. They include the following:

   - Join a self-help group.
   - Teach the assertiveness principles to others.
   - Maintain buddy contacts.
   - Join another group (not necessarily an assertiveness group).
   - Prepare for an unsympathetic environment.
   - Prepare for personal setbacks. Have back up coping statements ready for times when techniques do not work. For example, if you are backsliding say, "I slipped up but I've got the skills now."
   - Predict specific roadblocks you may face. What situations are likely to be most difficult in the future? Have a "road map" ready to handle those situations, which includes a plan of action, techniques you can use, and self-statements that would be helpful.
   - Keep a diary of successes and problem areas.
   - Periodically review the techniques you have learned and your notebook of handouts and assignments. Decide which ones could work for you.

2. Develop a specific, **realistic** plan including only those techniques you plan on using.

PURPOSE

By the end of this exercise you will have devised a personal transfer-of-change and maintenance plan.

EXERCISE

1. You should take several minutes to devise a plan.
2. Break into couples or pairs to discuss and refine plans.
3. Share plans with entire group.
4. Group helps evaluate the plan of each member. Is it complete? Realistic? How can group members help each other to maintain change?

Transfer of Change *(Continued)*

WHAT ARE YOUR MAINTENANCE PLANS FOR THE NEXT MONTH?

In relation to yourself? (e.g., "I will write down my self-talk whenever I get angry.")

_____

_____

_____

In relation to others? (e.g., " I will a set time each week to discuss problems with my partner.")

_____

_____

_____

WHAT ARE YOUR MAINTENANCE PLANS FOR THE NEXT YEAR?

In relation to yourself? (e.g., "I will practice relaxation every week so I will be ready.")

_____

_____

_____

In relation to others? (e.g., "I will encourage my partner to go out more, and will not be possessive.")

_____

_____

_____

Adapted from Wexler (1991) and Rose, Hanusa, Tolman, and Hall (1982), *A Group Leader's Guide to Assertiveness*.

Monthly Behavior Inventory

Name:_____ Date:_____

1. **MONTHLY SUCCESS.** Describe one way in the past month in which you successfully kept yourself from being aggressive or successfully used something you learned in group. The success can be large or small.

   Specifically, did you do any of the following?

   _____ Calmly stood up for my rights
   _____ Expressed my feelings appropriately
   _____ Told myself to relax
   _____ Changed my thoughts from negative to positive
   _____ Took a time-out

2. **PROBLEM SITUATION.** Describe a problem situation from the past month. What did you say or do specifically?

   How angry did you become?

1	10	20	30	40	50	60	70	80	90	100

   Not at   Extremely
   all angry   angry

3. **AGGRESSION.** Did you become verbally or physically aggressive toward anyone in the past month (including threats and damage to property)?

   Yes _____   No _____   If yes, what did you do?

   _____ Use of weapon   _____ Destruction of property
   _____ Slapping   _____ Choking
   _____ Kicking   _____ Sexual abuse
   _____ Punching   _____ Verbal abuse
   _____ Throwing things   _____ Emotional abuse
   _____ Threatening   _____ Other (explain): _____

   What would you do in a similar situation in the future to avoid becoming aggressive?

4. **HOMEWORK.** Did you complete Homework for the month?

   Yes _____   No _____   If yes, what did you do?

   Reviewed handouts?   Yes _____   No _____
   Completed assignment?   Yes _____   No _____
   Practiced exercise?   Yes _____   No _____
   Communicated with partner? Yes _____   No _____

© 1999 Springer Publishing Company.

Postcounseling Assessment Interpretation and Program Evaluation

OBJECTIVE

The objective of this assessment is to evaluate the counseling with a questionnaire, and the results can be compared to those prior to counseling.

POSTCOUNSELING QUESTIONNAIRE

Name _____   Client number _____

Group _____   Date _____

Counselors_____

Date that you entered counseling _____

Date that you left or completed counseling _____

Marital status while in the program:

| Married | _____ | Cohabitating | _____ | Separated _____ | Single_____ |

| Widowed | _____ | Divorced | _____ | Other: _____ |

Current marital status:

| Married | _____ | Cohabitating | _____ | Separated _____ | Single_____ |

| Widowed | _____ | Divorced | _____ | Other: _____ |

How long have you been in this relationship?

Years _____   Months _____   Don't know _____

Is this the same partner you had while you were in the program?

Yes_____   No _____   I'm not sure _____

What type of counseling format was used?

Men's Group _____ Family Counseling_____ Women's Group_____ Couples Group __

Couples Counseling_____   Individual Counseling_____

What kinds of counseling methods were used in your program?

Self-Esteem Enhancement	_____	Assertiveness Training	_____
Communication Skills	_____	Emotional Awareness Training	_____
Emotional Expression Training	_____	Problem-Solving Skills	_____
Anger Management	_____	Stress Management	_____
Explorations of Gender Roles	_____	Role Playing	_____
Tests/Evaluations	_____	Social History	_____
Support Outside Sessions (hotline, counselor access)	_____	Drug/Alcohol Intervention/ Treatment	_____
Building Social Support Systems	_____		

Postcounseling Assessment Interpretation and Program Evaluation *(Continued)*

Handout

How long were you in the program?   Months _____   Weeks _____

Did you finish the program? Yes _____   No _____

If you did not finish the program, what were your reasons?
   Did not feel it was effective _____
   Did not like the staff for the program _____
   Did not feel I needed it _____
   Time conflicted with job_____
   Other (Specify):_____

Was there violence or abuse while you were in the program?
   Yes _____   No_____

If yes, was it: Physical _____   Verbal _____   Sexual _____

If the violence was physical, compared to before you entered the program, was it?
   Less severe _____   About the same _____   More severe _____

If the abuse was verbal, compared to before you entered the program, was it?
   Less severe _____   About the same _____   More severe _____

If the abuse was sexual, compared to before you entered the program, was it?
   Less severe _____   About the same _____   More severe _____

Who was the abusive one?
   Yourself _____   Both _____   Partner _____

How often did the abuse occur?
   Once _____   Once a week_____   Once a month _____   2–3 times a week_____
   2–3 times a month _____   Daily _____   Other (Specify):_____

Did any of the techniques shown or talked about in the program help you deal more effectively
with your situation?
   Yes _____   No_____   Don't Know _____   Does Not Apply _____
   If yes, which ones?_____

How much has the program helped to overcome other problems besides the abuse?
   Not Very Helpful _____   Helpful _____   Fairly Helpful_____   Very Helpful_____

How would you rate the program?
   Very Poor ____   Poor ____   Good ____   Very Good ____   Excellent ____   Don't Know ____

Postcounseling Assessment Interpretation and Program Evaluation *(Continued)*

How would you rate the program staff?
    Very Poor ____ Poor ____ Good ____ Very Good ____ Excellent ____ Don't Know ____

Would you recommend this program to others? Yes _____ No _____

Do you think your counselors understood your specific problems?
    Yes _____ No _____ Don't Know _____

Have you ever been in counseling before? Yes _____ No _____

What factors influenced your decision to enter our counseling program?
_____
_____
_____

What in the program was most beneficial to you?
_____
_____
_____

In what ways do you think the program can be improved?
_____
_____
_____